A NOTE ON THE AUTHOR

JENNY DISKI was born in 1947 in London, where she lived most of her life. She was the author of ten novels, four books of travel and memoir, including *Stranger on a Train* and *Skating to Antarctica,* two volumes of essays and a collection of short stories. Her journalism appeared in publications including the *Mail on Sunday,* the *Observer* and the *London Review of Books,* to which she contributed more than two hundred articles over twenty-five years.

jennydiski.co.uk

In Gratitude
JENNY DISKI

BLOOMSBURY
LONDON · OXFORD · NEW YORK · NEW DELHI · SYDNEY

Bloomsbury Paperbacks
An imprint of Bloomsbury Publishing Plc

50 Bedford Square   1385 Broadway
London   New York
WC1B 3DP   NY 10018
UK   USA

www.bloomsbury.com

BLOOMSBURY and the Diana logo are trademarks of Bloomsbury Publishing Plc

First published in Great Britain 2016
This paperback edition first published in 2017

MIX
Paper from
responsible sources
FSC
www.fsc.org   FSC® C020471

To find out more about our authors and books visit www.bloomsbury.com. Here you will find
extracts, author interviews, details of forthcoming events and the option to sign up for our newsletters.

For Louis and Rosie with love

CONTENTS

FOREWORD

by Anne Enright

For Jenny Diski, writing, like smoking or seeking solitude, was just how she spent the day. It was a form
of thinking. She didn't seem to worry about the gap
between her brain and the page. And though she found
it hard to write her first novel, she was, by the middle of
her writing life, pretty much indifferent to the distinction between memoir, fiction, travelogue and review. 'It
is all "writing",' she said. This impatience with category
helped her to move out of the shadow of Doris Lessing,
the great fiction writer who took Diski in as a troubled
teenager, where she was impressed and overwhelmed by
all Lessing's clever, critical friends. Their dinner-table
conversation terrified her, especially when talking about
books or films: 'I couldn't understand how it was so
easy for them to have a point of view, to know how and
why things "worked".'

Shifting between genres helps a writer dodge judgement; it also confounds some sense of authority,
especially authority that proves disappointing or false.
Keep moving, keep talking; stay witty, precise, light on
your feet. As the grandchild of Jewish immigrants from
Russia and Poland, Diski didn't know 'where she was'
in London, being 'sort of Jewish and English', so the
discovery that she could move between genres made
some sense of that too, perhaps. But her restlessness

was more than geopolitical. As a girl she was moved from one house to another in order to protect her from useless and abusive parents, and she was, in these new spaces, always unsure of how to fit in. 'Was it OK to use this or that bathroom, which things were special to whom? I never knew the rules of each family or group, the systems, what is and isn't done in other people's houses and when.'

It was not just the invisible boundaries of English life that confused and interested Diski, or the boundaries in the houses of strangers where she was expected to live, but not to belong, Diski's own physical boundaries were ignored or breached at a very early age. It is hard to forget the image of her mother stroking between her teenage daughter's legs when they were reunited in a bedsitting-room in Brighton. Or the image of Diski as a young child, playing the usual game with her parents after a bath, 'running away from one, whose fingers tickled their way between my legs to my vulva, to the other, just a few feet across the room, gesturing at me, waiting impatiently to do the same thing'. This was the closest the three of them got to playing Happy Families, and though Diski recognises the 'torment' of the tickling, 'The adult me raises her eyebrows slightly, but makes no further comment.'

This slight lift of the brow is the option Diski chooses. Better than howling, perhaps. Certainly better than spending years in one mental institution or another (it didn't work, she says, nothing worked). It is her life – she can respond to it in any way she likes. The reader, meanwhile, reels back in incomprehension. What were they thinking? Diski does not tell us. She describes it as: 'the more or less unconscious behaviour of my parents towards me', and she forgives them, or seems to, in a way she could never manage to forgive Lessing. The need to understand can be an additional burden for the victim, though 'victim' is not one of Diski's words. It was not that bad, she says about her appalling parents. It was not that bad, she says about her first experience of sex at fourteen. 'I had no sense that I was especially violated by the rape', putting the quietness of her response down to the fact it happened in 1961. 'A different *zeitgeist*, luckily for me.'

Well, yes. The '*zeitgeist*' seeps into the body's interior, of course it does, and somatic experience changes with the language we use to describe it. (*Hysterica passio*, down!) But there must be some term for this kind of fallacy: if the world says you have not suffered, then you will not have suffered (luckily for you). It is not the man who hurt you, but making a fuss about the man, making a fuss about yourself. Sometimes, when I read Diski, I get a flash of real madness in there – by which I mean complete irrationality – and sometimes, or most of the time, I agree with every single word she says.

As so often with memoir, critics describe Diski as being free of embarrassment, probably because she writes with such clarity about shameful subjects like madness, poverty and bad sex. Diski did not fuss about the line between private and public: 'I've never had a sense that privacy has anything to do with people knowing things about you,' she said in an interview, though it is hard to think of another definition for the word. 'I start with me, and often enough end with me.' The world is not a problem because, on the page, the world and the self are both contained.

In fact Diski only describes sexual encounters in order to declare them uninteresting, and I find her work to be full of embarrassment, suffused with it, both for herself and others. 'He only shuffled on his knees across the room to ask if I would kiss him,' she says of a rabbi 'with Humbertian hankerings', who helped find her accommodation at the age of twelve. At fourteen, she was 'embarrassed into' having sex for the first time with a strange man who followed her in the street. Two years later, in Doris Lessing's care, despite the fact that she didn't have 'much interest in sex' she is sent to a gynaecologist for a Dutch cap. The doctor screams at her and she flees 'shaken and embarrassed', as well she might. Her desires have been ascribed and then denied by someone else, who then shouts that it is all her fault. This incident seems to sum up something for Diski, who makes it clear that she wanted nothing. In the circumstances, wanting nothing is the only possible choice.

More than fifty years later, when she receives a diagnosis of pulmonary fibrosis and lung cancer, Diski experiences 'Embarrassment, at first, to the exclusion of all other feelings'. What is there to be embarrassed about? This is not social unease so much as mortification; the shame that kills you or makes you laugh. Diski chooses the latter, of course. A few moments later, 'I got a joke in.'

Diski was, as a foundling child, always 'wrong'. She did not fit – except, on occasion, into some wonderful clothes – so there is a constant wriggling out from under embarrassment in the scenes she describes. She does not claim to be right, or in charge, but she does claim a seat at the table, she insists on her right to a point of view. Writing is where this happens and she was never so much at home as on the page. Her great facility with sentences left a slight anxiety about structure – the shape she found most natural, or available, was that of the essay and she thrived in the *London Review of*

Books, a place like Lessing's dinner table (but much better), where people say the most interesting things and women seldom complain.

It seems to work, this trick with the eyebrow. Pain is a bit of a blank, and though Diski loved blank spaces and sought them out – as in her trip to Antarctica – she also went there to generate words, to say what blankness is like. A writer with such an appreciation of nothing – who wants nothing, or would like to want nothing – is the best, most contradictory guide to the encroaching nothingness of death. Her final book is, in places, difficult and sad, but it is also full of gratitude for the way things turned out. Given the start she had in life, the end of it was amazing: productive, settled, full of love for her husband, the Poet, for her daughter and grandchildren, and all of this a surprise to her, all of it important. The pain and sadness she feels when she thinks about her husband's distress when she is dead is a 'mirroring of another soul'. This astonishing empathetic leap is, perhaps, 'an exercise in the reality of love'.

It is more than moving – this late love over which death has no dominion – it is a statement about how to be a proper human being. It also begs many questions about the kinds of love offered and withheld in her childhood. A terrible, small sadness runs through this book and it is not about being born to a couple of freaks, or about dying away from the people you cannot bear to lose. At the end of her life, Diski finally writes about the most difficult and inspiring relationship of her adult life. Before she goes, she turns to take one good, last look at Doris.

There is no answer here, there is only Diski's hurt and confusion, her endlessly circling sorrow. Why did Lessing want her as an object of charity, when she did not want her as a person, and what was wrong with Diski, that she could not bridge the gap?

In a way, their dysfunctions slotted together perfectly: the abandoned girl is taken in by an abandoning mother. Lessing left two children behind in Southern Rhodesia, when she left in 1949, taking with her her first finished manuscript and her third child, Peter, who was then two years old. A mother's love did not seem to do Peter much good, and Diski picks, fretfully, at his wasted life. He was, she wrote, a man who 'from nineteen had never worked or had a proper job, no real relation-ships, sexual or otherwise . . . who lived alone with his mother, lay on his bed when he wasn't watching television in the afternoon and evening and eventually became so gross, in the sense of fat and uncouth, that very few people could put up with it'. Diski could be a bit funny about people getting fat, it has to be said, but the rest of the description seems to hold true. There he is on YouTube, getting out of a black cab behind Doris, the day she is doorstepped with the news that she has won the Nobel Prize. He has a string of onions in one hand and a big globe artichoke in the other. They have been shopping, but Doris had the sense to bring a bag. The hand holding the artichoke is suspended in a grubby-looking sling. He is clearly eccentric. And Lessing's response to the news – fake dismay, dismissal, a little surge of glee – makes her seem eccentric too. Perhaps it was just genetic.

If not love, then literature – surely Lessing gave this brilliant girl the gift of books, and is this not the same thing? Diski made a life's work of what she learned in Charrington Street: a house bought on the proceeds of *The Golden Notebook*, when Lessing was at the height of her fame. Some mysterious theft or transference of writerly power must have happened at the kitchen table, over the boeuf stroganoff and Mateus Rosé.

The sad fact is that Lessing kept all the power for herself. She never owned to reading a book by Diski – who wrote seventeen books – but she had no compunction writing a novel based on her own experience. *Memoirs of a Survivor* is about a woman driven to a 'frenzy of irritation' by the foundling in her house, 'a self-presenting little *madam*', who, as Diski describes, 'spears passers-by and neighbours with her acid insights and cruel stories'. Diski is intrigued by this description of her teenage self, because it felt so different to be her; she reserves the right to remember her life from the inside. But the thing she really wants to talk about, in her last days, is not the books; it is the love she needed from Lessing, and did not get.

The gratitude of the title (or InGratitude – the pun was surely intended) is in part for the start this woman gave Diski, the inspirational circle of bohemian friends, the money, the work ethic and good advice. It is also gratitude for the love she found in later life – or stumbled upon, and had the wit to see. Happy endings are the hardest. Diski writes against the clock, like a woman knitting faster because she is running out of wool. In her last days, she rang her editor at the *London Review of Books* to say, 'She didn't think she could write anymore; she still had the words – and even the sentences – but they were no longer getting through to her fingers.' She was still writing in her head, she was still living in the words, she was still alive.

DIAGNOSIS

The future flashed before my eyes in all its preordained banality. Embarrassment, at first, to the exclusion of all other feelings. But embarrassment curled at the edges with a weariness, the sort that comes over you when you are set on a track by something outside your control, and which, although it is not your experience, is so known in all its cultural forms that you could unscrew the cap of the pen in your hand and jot down in the notebook on your lap every single thing that will happen and everything that will be felt for the foreseeable future. Including the surprises.

I got a joke in.

'So – we'd better get cooking the meth,' I said to the Poet, sitting to one side and slightly behind me. The Poet with an effort got his face to work and responded properly. 'This time we quit while the going's good.' The doctor and nurse were blank. When we got home the Poet said he supposed they didn't watch much US TV drama. It was only later that I thought that maybe, ever since *Breaking Bad*'s first broadcast, oncologists and their nurses all over the Western world have been subjected to the meth-cooking joke each time they have applied their latest, assiduously rehearsed, non-brutal techniques in 2014 for telling a patient as gently but honestly as possible, having first sized up their inner resilience with a few apparently innocent questions ('Tell me what you have been expecting from this appointment'), that they have inoperable cancer. Perhaps they failed to laugh at my – doubtless evasive – bid to lighten the mood, not because they didn't get the reference, but because they had said to each other too often after such an appointment: 'If I hear one more patient say they should start cooking meth, I'm going to wrestle them to the ground and bellow death into their faces – "Pay attention, I'm fucking telling you something important!"' I was mortified at the thought that before I'd properly started out on the cancer road, I'd committed my first platitude. I was already a predictable cancer patient.

Then again, what if I had taken the other option, and sat in dignified silence for a moment collecting myself, which I'm sure is how one would describe the short hiatus, and then asked serious, intelligent questions about the nature of the treatment the Onc Doc was suggesting, not to 'cure' me (he had slipped that in right at the start for me to run with or blank out, as I chose), but which had a 20 to 30 per cent chance of producing a remission for an unguessable period? After listening as carefully as my muddled head could manage to his answer (three cycles of chemotherapy, a scan, a course of radiotherapy, taking us up to Christmas, almost, then we would see), I would then be obliged to ask the next, inevitable 'how long' question, hedged about with all the get-out clauses for Onc Doc, who after all wasn't to blame for my cancer.

'Of course, I understand it would be unreasonable of me to expect you to know, with any certainty, when I'm likely to die if I have the treatment. I'm sure it's different for everyone, and only based on statistics, but could you perhaps give me a general idea: years . . . months . . . weeks?'

The print size in my mind decreased with time's incremental decline, and as I arrived at the last word – weeks – it suddenly struck me, with all the force of the fullest sense of the word 'struck', that this could actually be his answer and not just the logical next time period in my sentence. Every cell in my body, except those responsible for maintaining a reasonable, calm exterior, was now lindy-hopping at that possibility, the only one that hadn't occurred to me until that moment. Weeks. Still, the question itself was there waiting in line for me in the ready-made scripts file, for this unique to me but culturally familiar diagnostic moment, just after the Contemporary International Smart Cancer Joke.

Not that I've asked yet. I am getting ahead of myself. In fact, the Onc Doc, my Onc Doc as I now think of him, was drawing little circles, the results of my PET scan and bronchoscopy, on a ready-made outline map of a human torso, skinned and boned to show the lungs and lymph nodes, so that I could see the smallness of the tumour (good) in the lower left lobe, but also that it was too close to the pleura to be operable (not so good), and how its somewhat active cells (rather bad) had already travelled along two lymph nodes up to a third beside my oesophagus (more than rather bad). With that careful insertion of 'to treat, not to cure' in his suggested plan of action, he had in effect just told me I was going to die in his care, sooner rather than later. Now I had to decide, do I want to ask that obvious next question? And the one after that? (How long, then, without treatment?) I believe he knew exactly how these appointments went. Why should I make it easy for him? I now thought. It's quite hard to rapidly absorb the notion that someone forecasting your fairly imminent death might not be your enemy. More than that, the great weariness combined with the previously mentioned embarrassment, at the idea of asking question B or no. 2 and thereby setting the expected ball of clichés rolling, was overwhelming. Instead of complying, I imagined I could instead nod a thank you and take my leave of the doctor and the nurse. The Poet would leave with me, and we'd never mention it again. The Woman with No Name approach. A short shriek of Morricone, after the door has closed behind us. But that wouldn't do, either. After the heroic moment there would be the hour-by-hour living. Everyday life, even a shortened one, doesn't permit heroic blankness in the way film does. Say, Leone's long, long close-up of Eastwood's or Fonda's impassive face; the Warhol movie of John Giorno sleeping for five hours and twenty minutes; Jarman's seventy-nine-minute single shot of saturated blue.

Or I could do nothing. I could sit in sadistic silence waiting for whatever is next on his list of diagnostic appointment moves for all occasions.

'Yes? And?'

Sullen rudeness is a possible option handed to us cancerees. It would institute a period of bad behaviour as one's own private glumly-gleeful saturnalia, world turned upside down, lord-of-misrule regulated havoc, for a short period before the great slog of getting on with it began again, cancer or no cancer. I probably couldn't sulk unto death, no matter that I'm one of the foremost sulkers on the planet. I'd get hungry. Or want to watch TV. Or even have an itch I had to scratch, and any such desire immediately and fatally cracks the implacable wall of sulk. Another route through the carefully tended maze of standard responses looks like the most spontaneous, although it really needs to be yelled by Jack Lemmon, tortoise-style, sticking his neck right out, inches from

Onc Doc's face. 'You're telling me I've got CANCER? That I'm going to DIE, because don't think I don't know that INOPERABLE means it'll spread along the tracks from lymph node to nymph load.' (I'd apologise for that, but I'm not sorry.) 'You've just said you reckon, with all your hedging and ditching, that I'm going to be DEAD IN THREE YEARS. If I'm LUCKY. Have I got that RIGHT?'

Actually, he said 'two to three years' with treatment. (The 'weeks' moment passed, leaving me less cheered than I ought to have been.) But I've taken the long view to stop any quibbling. I do wonder, now he's laid the numbers out, with all the ifs and buts and maybes, how he manages his probability predictions. Does he pop an extra year on after 'or', for luck, like one for the pot? Or does he shift the lower end of the prediction a little towards the future to soften the felt brevity of a single year to someone whose time is slipping past at the speed of a sixty-seven-year-old's perception. Perhaps he's always as scrupulously accurate as possible in these situations, because, although he would like to offer a false glimmer of optimism which is said to be as good as a placebo, he doesn't want to risk my ghostly or my of-kin's litigious fury if I died a day short of his over-generous soonest prediction. So I should believe him because fear of a lawsuit makes doctors realistic and therefore trustworthy. This not crazily short but vague two-to-three-years is a difficult real-life calculation for me. On the one hand, to die pushing seventy years of age is no great tragedy, even if my id would like to know what the fuck age has got to do with being rubbed out. Even so, such reasonableness doesn't take account of the kind of thoughts that run swiftly through my mind. Two to three years. Will the battery on the TV remote run out first? How many inches will the weeping birch grow, the one planted by the Poet for my sixtieth birthday (soppy old radical versifier)? I suppose I won't need another cashmere sweater to keep me warm come the planet's apocalypse, the ones I've already got will survive the moths for a couple of years or even three should it come sooner than my own apocalypse. I very much regret the disappearance of a website I once bookmarked called 'Sensible Units'. It took a scientific unit of quantity and resolved it into units that are much more easily or entertainingly imagined. Who knew that 1 cm of depth is equivalent to 29 human female fingernail thicknesses? Or that 80 gigabytes can be visualised as 110 CDs or 25 human genomes? So, when my Onc Doc announced that I had cancer, inoperable cancer, and that there was no cure, but some lengthy and famously unpleasant treatment that might get in the way of its speedy (the word 'aggressive' comes to mind but wasn't actually said) progress, I chose the threadbare joke, from the already ready possible options. Because I had to choose something. But, as well as doing what I had to do in my new role, and for more than any other reason, it was a short-term panic-stricken solution for the flood of embarrassment, much more powerful than alarm or fear, that engulfed and mortified me at finding myself set firmly on that particular well-travelled road. I am and have always been embarrassed by all social rituals that require me to participate in a predetermined script. It may simply be that I am not a natural actor. That would account for the funk. Perhaps, having been handed this inescapable part, I was suffering from stage fright. It goes deep. I can perform at other people's dinner tables like a chattering magpie, arguing and picking up on the conversation to make a joke or say something smart.

Then I go home covered with a layer of self-disgust as if I'd been rolling in donkey shit, and for a day or two afterwards, I stay in bed with the covers over my head in shame. In public and prescribed ritual, I have no easy get-out, but I can't just get on with it. The only way I can manage – gracelessly – is to keep my head down, my eyes low, dig my fingers hard into my palm and move my mouth a little, like John Redwood singing the Welsh national anthem, while other people enjoy themselves intoning the required utterances. Ever since I was a child, it's been like that.

'You have to say, "I wish you long life," and shake his hand,' my father told me on our way to visit a relative sitting shiva. The rest of the journey was an agony of anticipation. I knew I couldn't say those words. I wouldn't be able to get them out. They were ridiculous, not what I'd really ever say to someone else. Not what small children would say and do, and it seems I could only play one role at a time. I've never been able to make my face work properly while repeating a set speech. Also, it seemed mean-spirited towards the newly dead to hope the mourner lived longer, who after all already had. 'It's what you do. Just say it and then go and get a smoked salmon bagel.' I could almost see that the anguish of the occasion was not actually mine, but belonged to the bereaved. Still, I couldn't bear to think about doing it. It wasn't what I would say, therefore I couldn't say it. I think also, it was expected of me, and therefore I couldn't do it. I wonder what would have happened if I hadn't been instructed. Would I have taken his hand and said something suitable? What could that be? I might just have said, as I would now, 'I'm very sorry.' Why wasn't I allowed to do that? Because. We arrived and I took the hand offered me, but failed to look into his eyes, which, because of the low seating arrangement for chief mourners, were level with mine. I think I stared off to one side. And I managed only a mumbled noise, a strangled moan. Nothing that could be mistaken for 'I wish you long life.' I'd failed and although I knew I was in trouble, I was relieved not to have said the words out loud, while people watched me and smiled at the sweet little girl maintaining the grown-up tradition with archaic words translated from the Yiddish.

Growing up hasn't helped. Marriage ceremonies have been as difficult, even though I was an adult. The first was a blur, although I remember the fingers digging into my palm, and handing over my gold opal ring to my betrothed, just before we went in to be 'done', so he could slip it on my finger with the opal at the back, because we hadn't got round even to thinking about a ring until the morning of the registry office ceremony. Certainly, I was embarrassed and tied in knots by the corniness of the whole performance. Roger didn't mind, he always enjoyed me disconcerting his parents. By the time of my second marriage, well into my dog days, I had enough confidence to ask the registrar who was to perform the ceremony if I could just say 'Yes' when it got to the bit where I was required to say 'I do', and to miss out repeating the affirmations about better or worse, sickness and blah-blah-blah, already much minimised by me and the Poet. She looked at me as if I'd kicked her favourite bunny. 'We are allowed to give people permission to do that,' she said. 'But only when they're terminally ill and have difficulty speaking.' I stopped myself from saying that I wasn't feeling too perky, actually, and who knows what it might turn into. Properly shamed, I went through with it, sotto voce and choking back some but not all the nervous giggles that always rise up when I'm forced to participate in ritual. The Poet said I behaved childishly and I completely agreed. I decided I was definitely not going to do that again, no matter how practical it might be.

Now I was faced with the prospect of a rather lengthy (in one view) public/private performance by which to be excruciated. A sudden death requires others to deal with the difficulty of ritual. A stroke, a heart attack. Then it's all someone else's problem. But this diagnostic appointment was the announcement of yet another version of the show going on the road in which I was to star. I had been formally inducted into Cancer World. (Mixing my metaphors, I'm afraid. Which should it be, the theme park or the lack of variety show?) I was handed my script, though all the lines were known already and the moves were paced out. There are no novel responses possible. Absolutely none that I could think of. Responses to the diagnosis; the treatment and its side effects; the development of cancer symptoms; the pain and discomfort; the dying; the death. Do I have to start a campaign? Wear a badge, run, climb walls, swim inordinate lengths, dance the tango for a very long time, in return for money for cancer research? Whatever that is. Does the money go to the drug companies? To university labs? To Jeremy Hunt? What is this crowd-funded research, where is it happening? Am I going to appear calm in the face of destiny? Actually cheerful, with people saying I was wonderful? Should I affirm my atheism or collapse into religious comfort? Or should I turn my face to the wall? And when the symptoms kick in, will I suffer in silence, quote Epictetus and Marcus Aurelius, or will I refuse to go gentle and make an almighty fuss ('Excuse me, I'm the cancer patient here!'). Dear God, not a bucket list?

Really, there is nothing that I want to do before I die, except perhaps just lie back and enjoy the morphine, daydreaming my way to oblivion.

One thing I state as soon as we're out of the door: 'Under no circumstances is anyone to say that I lost a battle with cancer. Or that I bore it bravely. I am not fighting, losing, winning or bearing.' I will not personify the cancer cells inside me in any form. I reject all metaphors of attack or enmity in the midst, and will have nothing whatever to do with any notion of desert, punishment, fairness or unfairness, or any kind of moral causality. But I sense that I can't avoid the cancer clichés simply by rejecting them. Rejection is conditioned by and reinforces the existence of the thing I want to avoid. I choose how to respond and behave, but a choice between doing this or that, being this or that, really isn't freedom of action, it's just picking one's way through an already drawn flow-chart. They still sit there, to be taken or left, the flashing neon markers on the road that I would like to think isn't there for me to be travelling down. I am appalled at the thought, suddenly, that someone at some point is going to tell me I am on a journey. I try but I can't think of a single aspect of having cancer, start to finish, that isn't an act in a pantomime in which my participation is guaranteed however I believe I choose to play each scene. I have been given this role. (There, see? Instant victim.) I have no choice but to perform and to be embarrassed to death. I wish you long life.

We'd hardly got home before I said: 'Well, I suppose I'm going to write a cancer diary.' The only other thing I might have said was: 'Well, I'm not going to write a cancer diary.' Right there: a choice? I'm a writer, have been since I was small, and have earned my living at it for thirty years. I write fiction and non-fiction, but it's almost always personal. I start with me, and often enough end with me. I've never been apologetic about that, or had a sense that my writing is 'confessional'. What else am I going to write about but how I know and don't know the world? I may not make things up in fiction, or tell the truth in non-fiction, but documentary or invented, it's always been me at the centre of the will to put descriptions out into the world. I lie like all writers but I use my truths as I know them in order to do so.

'I wonder if I am not talking yet again about myself. Shall I be incapable, to the end, of lying on any other subject?' I used this quote from *Malone Dies* as the epigraph to my non-fiction so-called travel book *Skating to Antarctica*, though it would have been apt, to my mind, at the front of any book I've written, fiction or non-fiction, memoir or travel, history or fantasy. *Skating* concerned a voyage I took around the Antarctic peninsula and the story of my rather brief, rackety relationship with my mother. 'You know,' I'd say gaily to people who asked what it was about. 'Icebergs, mothers. That sort of thing.' I couldn't even describe the most extraordinary landscape on the planet without reference to myself and my life outside the Antarctic cruise. I can't use my eyes to see things without my eyes knowing that what they see is conditioned by what I've known and what I've been. Ditto my mind to think things. So be it. I'm a writer. I've got cancer. Am I going to write about it? How am I not? I pretended for a moment that I might not, but knew I had to, because writing is what I do and now cancer is what I do, too. And then the weariness. A fucking cancer diary? Another fucking cancer diary. I think back to cancer diaries I have read, just because they're there. You don't seek cancer diaries out, they come at you as you turn the pages of magazines and newspapers or thumb through Twitter and blogs. How many have I read? I can't remember, but they've spanned decades. I recall Ruth Picardie, a young woman in her thirties, with small children. John Diamond, married to Nigella Lawson and dying stylishly. Ivan Noble, a BBC science and technology writer; Tom Lubbock, art critic; Susan Sontag, although not exactly a diary, mined her cancer for a famous essay about the cultural nature of illness. Those stood out, they were all professional writers and most wrote their diaries as occasional or regular series for newspapers or online blogs. Can there possibly be anything new to add? Isn't the cliché of writing a cancer diary going to be compounded by the impossibility of writing in it anything other than what has already been written, over and over? Same story, same ending. Weariness. The odd thing is, narcissistic writer though I am, I have always thought of writing straight autobiography as incredibly tedious. I couldn't put hand to keyboard without there being something else, some other component in the narrative than just my personal history. In 1984, while I was in a deep and long depression, largely, I think, about how I wasn't being a writer, my previously adoptive or foster mother, Doris Lessing, would say, in her matter-of-fact, impatient way: 'Well, just write down your life story. It's interesting enough, and there are editors who can deal with sorting out your sentences and that kind of thing.' She wafted her arm in the air to show me how easy it would be. It was intended to encourage me. It made me even more silent with despair. I wasn't interested in just being published. I wasn't even interested in writing something 'interesting enough'. I was a writer and I couldn't understand why I wasn't writing. The answer was, I think, that I hadn't understood how writing gathers everything into itself to make a satisfactory piece. My story, someone else's story, a place, an idea, a dream, human anatomy, the mind acting on the world, vice versa, some or all and more yet unthought of, had to be combined in the right amounts in order to make a book, an essay, fiction, non-fiction, history, comedy, whatever, work. I was enough of a writer to know that writing the story of my interesting childhood was not being a writer. I was enough of a writer to be dismayed that Doris, having known me by then for nearly two decades, didn't know that about me. I was also, in spite of my depression, quite insulted that she thought my sentences needed such tending.

In my experience, writing doesn't get easier the more you do it. But there is a growth of confidence, not much, but a nugget, like a pearl, like a tumour. You learn that there is a process, and that it doesn't very much matter what you write, but how you do it, that is crucial, and that nothing I wrote, or you wrote, is ever going to be the same as what she wrote and he wrote, unless, as Truman Capote said, what you're dealing with isn't writing, but typing. So I've got cancer. I'm writing.

PART ONE

Doris and Me

My experience with death has been minimal and to varying degrees distant. I have never been in the presence of anyone when they died. The likely ones, family deaths, the deaths of my father and mother, are remote in space and time. My father died when I was nineteen, somewhere else, and I was told of it by phone. In the case of my mother I didn't even know she had died in the 1980s until my daughter Chloe found out eight years later. Between late 2010 and early 2011 there were two deaths: one a very elderly, long-time friend Joan Rodker, and the other, sudden and tragic, a couple of months later, my first husband, father of my daughter and my oldest friend, Roger. Then, during the final quarter of 2013, there were two more deaths within a month of each other, neither of them really unexpected after years of frailty, but both, Doris Lessing and her son Peter, having attachments of some complexity to each other, to my daughter and to me, going back even before I went at fifteen to live in their house.

When she died in November at the age of ninety-four, I'd known Doris for fifty years. In all that time, I've never managed to figure out a designation for her that properly and succinctly describes her role in my life, let alone my role in hers. We have the handy set of words to describe our nearest relations: mother, father, daughter, son, uncle, aunt, cousin, although that's as far as it usually goes in contemporary Western society.

Doris wasn't my mother. I didn't meet her until she opened the door of her house in Charrington Street, north of King's Cross, after I had knocked on it to be allowed in to live with her. What should I call her to others? For several months I lived with Doris, and worked in the office of a friend of hers. Then, after some effort, she persuaded my father to allow me to go back to school. As a punishment, he had vetoed further schooling after I was expelled – for climbing out of the first-floor bathroom window to go to a party in the town – from the progressive, co-ed boarding school that Camden Council had sent me to some years before. ('We think you will be better living away from your mother for some of the time. Normally, we would send you to one of our schools for maladjusted children, but because your IQ is so high, we're going to send you to a private school, St Christopher's, which takes a few local author-ity cases like yours,' the psychologists at University College Hospital had said to me, rather unpsycho-logically. I was eleven.) My father relented and Doris sent me to a progressive day school.

At the new school, aged 15 as I tried to ease myself back into being a schoolgirl after my adventures in real life (working full time in a shoe shop, a grocery shop, and then being a patient in a psychiatric hospital), I discovered I had to have some way of referring to the person I lived with to my classmates. It turned out that teenagers constantly refer to and complain about their parents and they use the regular handles. Not that I would, under the circumstances, have complained. But could I refer to Doris as my adoptive mother? She hadn't adopted me, although she'd suggested it. We even went to see a solicitor in the first month, who must have had a wilful teenager of his own, because instead of coolly discussing the legal situation, he turned to me and ranted about the awfulness of teenagers these days, my undeserved good fortune, the selfishness of giving my parents so much worry and his inability to believe I had any psychological problems – I merely wanted special treatment and attention. I stared at him, feeling both slapped and in the middle of someone else's cartoon, but before he could finish what sounded uncannily like the solicitor's speech in John Osborne's play *Inadmissible Evidence*, a year or so later, Doris grabbed my sleeve and we escaped down the winding wooden staircase, with the sound of his voice echoing behind us. In addition, my mother had one of her screaming fits and threatened to sue Doris for alienation of affection (hilarity ensued) if she tried to adopt me. So that was quietly dropped. I sometimes said 'adoptive mother' anyway, as an easy though inexact solution. It wasn't only for form's sake that it mattered how I referred to her; whenever I was called on to say 'Doris, my, er . . . sort of, adoptive mother . . . my, er . . . Doris . . .' to refer to my adult-in-charge, I was aware of giving the wrong impression.

For some reason, being precise, finding a simple possessive phrase that covered my situation, was very important. I didn't want to lie and I did want to find some way of summing up my circumstances accurately to others. But I hadn't been an adopted child. Both my parents were still alive and (regrettably, in my view) in contact with me. The changeover in my caretakers ('my caretaker'?) didn't happen until I was at an age when some had left school and gone to work, as I had after my expulsion from St Christopher's, until I ran away from my father in Banbury and went to stay with my mother in Hove, in her very small, one-bed bedsitting-room. That had lasted only a few days before the wisest move seemed to be to take what remained of my mother's Nembutal, lie down neatly on the bed and wait to die. 'How can you do this to me? Why can't you be decent, like other children?' she screamed when she found me. The night before in the bed we shared she had reached around my back, which was turned to her, and begun to caress my vulva. When I protested, she said: 'What's the matter? There's nothing wrong. I'm your mother. You're still my little girl.'

It was deemed a good idea to keep me away from my parents, so they popped me into the Lady Chichester Hospital in Hove. It was a small psychiatric unit in a large detached house, consisting mostly of young people, though none as young as I was. I became the official baby-of-the-bin, and both staff and patients looked after me and tried to shield me from the worst of the outbreaks of other people's madness. I, of course, was fascinated and felt quite at home and well cared for at last. The weekly fifteen minutes with the therapist was always the same.

'Is there anything you want to talk about?'

'Uh, no.'

After a few weeks of this I became convinced that the shrink knew something I didn't. He couldn't simply have meant what he said. The only thing I could think of was that I was pregnant, which, although I had only had sex with one man, several months before, I decided must be the case. I developed a secret terror that I was miraculously with child and the doctor was waiting for me to come to terms with it, though I never spoke of it to him. Apart from that, I wasn't mad at all and they weren't trying to treat me. I stayed there for four months, without medication, spending long periods sitting on the beach in Hove, staring at the sea – it was a winter of unprecedented ice and snow – while they tried to figure out what to do with me. After, for some reason, hankering for a job as a lab assistant, for which, of course, I was unqualified, I was eventually taken on by the Oxford Street department store Bourne and Hollingsworth as a sales assistant, an offer I was advised by Dr Watt, the psychiatrist in charge, to accept, because B&H had a hostel in London for its employees. But before that plan could be put into action, I received a letter from Doris Lessing, saying that although I didn't know her, she knew about me from her son, who had been in my class at St Christopher's. Much over-excited gossip, you can imagine, had been going on there about the wicked Jennifer Simmonds who'd got expelled and was now in a madhouse. The previous holder of the title of wickedest girl in the school had been Fanny Hill (*sic*), daughter of the historian, and mischievous child-namer, Christopher Hill.

Over the years I called Doris 'the woman I live with', which I worried could be taken to have something a little unseemly or suggestive about it in those not quite yet permissive days; 'the woman whose house I live in' (less unseemly but odd); or most often, 'Doris, my mumble, mumble, mumble', 'the person who blah-blah-blah'. Or I took a deep breath and went the whole hog: 'Doris, who invited me to go and stay at her house when she heard . . .' But with that the conversation was scuppered and once again, I'd end up telling the whole convoluted tale, which fairly rapidly, since Doris had also sent me to the Tavistock Adolescent Clinic to get 'sorted out', had become very boring, like a straight-forward writing down of my life story. For a while, I decided on 'foster mother' but the 'mother' part of it made me cringe (as it certainly made Doris cringe), and a friend, who wasn't English and didn't know about the system of care for children, objected that it made her sound as if she had taken me in for money. So taking account of cultural understandings, another possible designation hit the dust. I occasionally tried a light-hearted 'my benefactor', which had a theatrical and comic edge to it, but once again required a story to be told. There was 'my friend, Doris' but that didn't convey the dynamics of the relationship or the age discrepancy. 'My fairy godmother' was kept for those occasions when I was needing to end a conversation for my lack of interest in it. 'Auntie Doris' always got a laugh from Doris, and I think she suggested it as a joke when the matter came up. The name thing was an ongoing problem. Sometimes, for lack of a solution, I thought I'd simply call her 'my mother', but that made me so inordinately uncomfortable, 'mother' and 'my' being more than doubly cringeworthy, that even now I feel the need to reiterate that she wasn't really my mother. We never spoke about it in more detail than the Auntie Doris joke, but she must have had a sense of it because when my daughter was about a month old and lying on the carpet in her flat, Doris said, out of the blue, in the awkward, clipped and embarrassed tone she used for any discussion of our relationship, which I very well recognised by then: 'Do you want her to call me *Grandma*? Or some sort of thing like that?' I took it for the kindly and difficult gesture it was, but awkward and embarrassed myself by her manner, I said I thought 'Doris' would be the best name to call her. In any case, I said, 'She's got two grandmothers, even if one is invisible – please god.' I was quite taken by surprise at the thought that all along while I was trying to figure out how to refer to Doris, I actually had a real mother to call my own. But having thought that, it seemed irrelevant.

As with my cancer diagnosis, it's hard to avoid thundering clichés when writing about the start of my relationship with Doris, and hard not to make it sound either Dickensian or uncannily close to the fairy tales we have in the back of our minds. 'It's like something out of a fairy story' was a phrase people often said to me when they learned how I got to live with Doris. To which I would answer yes, or sort of, or say nothing at all. Or if I had the will, I would say something to the effect that the Cinderella fairy story of Doris and me was a rare instance of life after the ellipsis at the end of most fairy stories. *And they lived happily ever after.* People usually didn't much like that answer, because it messed up the simplicity of the story, and reminded them that Doris was not a handsome prince, nor I the foundling whose innate nobility was recognised by a prince of the true blood.

Still, it was close enough to the old tales. I was a sort of foundling. I was sort of recognised as or was elevated to being worthy of attention. I did proceed into another life. Or at least into a life that was probably different from the one I might have had if Doris had not issued her invitation and I'd remained on the Bourne and Hollingsworth path. Doris would have said firmly 'completely different'. Her view of the upshot of the B&H move was clear: she didn't think the chances of my survival very high. She even referred to me in interviews (in spite of our 'I won't talk about you if you don't talk about me' pact) as a waif whom she had rescued, and she frequently told me and others that, had I gone to the London hostel and a job as a salesgirl, I would not have become a writer, or even a managing director of B&H, but would have ended up pregnant and stuck with a child in an awful marriage (in that order), or pregnant and dead (in that order), or pregnant and a drug addict and dead (in any order – they were synonymous). She was adamant that I would have been dead before I was out of my teens. Being pregnant, married and/or a junkie represented *no life* to Doris. In fact, in relation to me and other young women, she considered that 'pregnant' and 'married' were alternative terms for 'death'. Only years later, when a challenging psychoanalyst queried the standard story, which I had thoroughly introjected, did I come to think that I would have had *some* life, *a* life, had Doris not intervened, which would still have been my own.

In his letter to Doris from St Christopher's after I was expelled (there were four of us, felled with one blow) and 'locked up' in the madhouse, her son Peter wondered, in all innocent generosity since we had by no means got on with each other at school, if, since I was 'quite intelligent', they might not be able to help me somehow. A few years later, Doris gave me Peter's letter. In fact, the Lady Chichester Hospital was no hellhole, and was for people who were more neurotic than mad. They were simply parking me while trying to find something to do with me that would keep me away from both of my unsatisfactory parents. Doris said in her letter to me that she had just moved into her first house, that it had central heating (she was particularly proud of that) and a spare room, so I might like to stay there, and perhaps, in spite of my father's reluctance, go back to school to get my exams and go to university. It wasn't clear in the letter how long I was invited to stay for, but the notion of going to university suggested something long-term, because I'd never heard of anyone going to university without having somewhere to live during the vacations.

I read the letter many times. The first time with a
kind of shrug: 'Ah, I see. That's what's going to happen
to me next.' Unexpected things had happened to me
so frequently and increasingly during my childhood
that they seemed normal. I came to expect them
with a Micawber-like passivity. Then I read the letter
again with astonishment that I did, after all, have a
fairy godmother. Then fear. Then a certain amount of
disappointment, and some real thought about whether
to accept or not, because I was excited about starting a new grown-up life in London as a salesgirl in
Oxford Street, in a *hostel*: girl things, make-up, cama-
raderie, misbehaviour, advice. Like boarding school or
the friendly psychiatric community I was already quite
contentedly in, but with pay and without pills. And
finally all these responses melded together like all the
colours of plasticine making grey sludge, and I had no
idea how to respond either to my own fears and expectations, or to this stranger for her invitation. So Doris
was not my mother. And aside from awkward social
moments, what she was to me was laid aside along with
other questions best left unthought.

The child was left with me in this way. I was in the
kitchen and, hearing a sound, went into the living
room, and saw a man and a half-grown girl standing
there. I did not know either of them, and advanced
with the intention of clearing up a mistake. The
thought in my mind was that I must have left my front
door open. They turned to face me. I remember how I
was even then, and at once, struck by the bright hard
nervous smile on the girl's face. The man – middle-
aged, ordinarily dressed, quite unremarkable in every

way – said: 'This is the child.' He was already on the way out. He had laid his hand on her shoulder, had smiled and nodded to her, was turning away.

I said: 'But surely . . .'

'No, there's no mistake. She's your responsibility.'

He was at the door. 'But wait a minute . . . '

'She is Emily Cartwright. Look after her.' And he had gone.

'Emily's you, of course,' Doris told me, handing me the final draft manuscript of *The Memoirs of a Survivor* in 1973. She always let me know when I appeared in her books, or when she used something I'd told her about, events from my past or present. She also told me who the other characters were. Not all of them had familiar real-world models, but many of the key characters in her stories and novels did, even some of the science fiction and fantasy ones. By the time she published *The Memoirs of a Survivor* the following year, I had been back in the bin, two different ones in London. Another book, *Briefing for a Descent into Hell*, published in 1971, centred on the story of my relationship with one of the other patients in St Pancras, while the later book, *Memoirs*, concerned, in part, not just a dramatisation of my arrival at Doris's, but also a fairly accurate and equally dramatic account of the time in my life, in the early 1970s, when Roger and I ran an 'alternative' school for some local kids, who had been persistently truanting and running wild, and were now threatened with being taken into care. Some of the later books had minor characters and odd events that were me and mine, but *Memoirs* and *Briefing* sit on my shelves quietly filled with Doris's take on me, and aspects of my life, reinterpreted for fiction. I only read each of them once, in manuscript. Until now, they've been patiently bearing my sideways glance, waiting for me to take another look, and to think about what I think about them, in terms of my real life and also in terms of fiction, and all the ways in which writers, including me, quite legitimately appropriate bits and pieces of lives and people for their own ends. The writer in me never had much trouble with the books that Doris solemnly indicated had characters who were 'you', and I felt only mildly aggrieved at her use of some of my best stories. After all, however convinced I was that I *was* a writer, I hadn't ever finished anything I started of my own writing. The sound of the voice in my ear as I typed, repeating 'This is crap, this is crap,' ensured that everything ended up in the waste-paper basket. So I had no real claim on my stories. And then, once I began writing myself, I realised it didn't matter what Doris might have done with those stories (her stories, once she wrote them), they were still available to me to do with as I wanted.

Before her invitation letter to me, Doris had an exchange of letters with Dr Watt in which he was extremely cautious, appearing to be worried about litigation from my parents, and perhaps from Doris, if he said anything too definite about them, or me, or too positive about Doris's plan, but essentially giving her the go-ahead. She was also visited by my father, the woman he lived with, Pam, and, my bête noire, Janet, Pam's daughter, a few years older than me and a prissy girl who told on me when she found me smoking in my room. My father, apparently and not surprisingly, tried to flirt with Doris and when that didn't seem to be working, to impress her with his knowledge of literature, which was less than very slight. Doris, in a follow-up letter to me, told me about it; she said that my father was preposterous, but she could handle him. Pam sat as she always did with her lips tightly pressed together and pursing them in and out with disapproval every time my name was spoken, and Janet piped up that I was so awful, and as an example, I had even wanted to go on the Aldermaston March with all those dirty beatniks. Not a good move, since Doris was a regular on the march herself.

Then it was all settled, although my father was adamant that I had to be punished for being expelled by not being allowed to go back to school. I'd had the two letters from Doris, and I replied thanking her for giving me such a wonderful opportunity (I did say that it was like a fairy story) and promising not to be any trouble, but warning her to ignore my father's accusations. He would, I was sure, tell her that I was wicked and worst of all a smoker, which I was but I'd stop if she wanted me to. It was this letter, Doris told me later, as did some friends of hers she spoke to at the time, that convinced her she was doing the right thing. It was intelligent (that again), humorous and well written. She was sure after reading it that having me in the house would work out, though I don't think it was clear in her mind any more than mine how long that was to be for.

So sometime in late February or March 1963, my mother and I took the train from Brighton to Victoria and then the Underground to Mornington Crescent (yes, really) and the ten-minute walk from the station to the street where Doris had bought her first house. It was opposite a concrete-and-glass boys' secondary modern school, and the houses on the other side were in the very early stages of gentrification. Most of them were quite dingy from the outside, council-owned houses rented to low-income families. Doris was one of the first to buy quite cheaply into the potential of the Georgian three-storeyed terraced houses, with their long, elegant windows and steps up to the front door. Black, I think. I knocked on the door, wearing an awful mustard-yellow woollen coat with a brown velvet collar and kind of pleated below a dropped waistline, which my mother thought was very grown-up and respectable, and which I would never wear again.

Doris answered the door with a small kitten in her arms.

'Look,' she said. 'She can be your cat. Some friends of mine got her, but they have no idea how to look after a cat. They were feeding her on lobster soup. She's called Grey Cat. Come in.' She was polite and I thought rather shy. She was in fact nervous at this first encounter with my mother, who Dr Watt had warned her was 'a very difficult lady'. It was lunchtime, and she had made soup for us, rather than for Grey Cat. It was a recipe she made often, with Campbell's chicken soup and an added tin of sweetcorn. My mother and I sat on the bench Doris had had built along one side of her kitchen table, while she sat on the other side on a chair, with access to the stove. I thought she hadn't finished doing up the house, and I was rather downhearted at the untidy state of the kitchen, the surfaces covered with glass jars and tins waiting for shelving that never got round to being built, the uncurtained window, and especially the bare floorboards which, being a lower-middle-class child of East End Jews, I thought were waiting for lino or tiles to be laid over them, rather than being fashionable bare boards waiting only for a final sanding. It didn't seem at all the sort of respectable place my mother would approve of, and I heard my mother in me deploring it and the owner who allowed it to be seen by visitors in its slovenly state. But very soon, along with my discarded coat, the chaotic kitchen seemed to be a proof of my entry into another kind of living altogether and one that I thought I might get the hang of if I paid attention.

I liked the soup, but have no recollection of the conversation. Doris said that my mother had done all the talking. She complained about my father's treatment of her, my treatment of her and the awful life she had come from in her miserable childhood and was now plunged back into. The shame of living on the dole in one room and the added shame of having an ungrateful daughter who behaved so badly she was put in a mental hospital, and now was going to be taken in by a stranger, who, she warned Doris, shouldn't herself be taken in by me. 'I'm the one who should be given a new home and looked after,' Doris told me my weeping mother had said. I don't remember, but it sounded like her. I imagine I was suffering my usual excruciating embarrassment when my mother had a meltdown in public. Doris said later that she'd felt sorry for the poor woman who was so disappointed by life, but she could only take on one of us, and that one was me. After a couple of hours, Doris eased my mother, still complaining about me, still crying about my father and her dreadful life, out of the house, and then, since it was term time and Peter was away at St Christopher's, Doris and I were left alone to figure out how we were to get on with each other.

———

A few years ago, someone asked how it came about that I ended up living with Doris Lessing in my teens. I was in the middle of the story of the toing and froing between my parents and was finally reaching the psychiatric hospital bit when the man said something extraordinary, something that had never occurred to me or to anyone else to whom I'd told the story.

'Why didn't you just do what you were told?' he asked.

I was lost for words. Although he sounded baffled rather than challenging, he was the sort of age a headmaster or my parents might have been when I was a teenage girl, and his question, and the tone of voice in which he asked it, might have come from their exasperation with me back then. The story so far had included quite a lot of me implicitly not doing as I was told, but there were also many times when no one told me what to do, and I had to make it up as I went along (nothing came with instructions). From the vantage point of children who did what they were told, in much the same way that soldiers followed orders, it was probably hard to imagine the outlawed wasteland where no one had any idea what they should do either before they did it or once they'd done it, or the badlands where a child might know as well or better than an adult what needed to be done. The question 'Why didn't you do what you were told?' had the charm for me of *Little Women* or *The Secret Garden*, or the novels of Noel Streatfeild, where even when things went awry there was always a neat and tidy family solution to set the whatevertheyarecalleds back on their path of contentment. I was confounded by the question he put to what was left of the insolent child inside me. Doing what I was told simply didn't have a place in my story of myself. It was perfectly clear that no one had any idea what to do, so they couldn't very well tell me. And that to do as I was told would have been to listen to people who were completely out of their depth, without a clue what to do except wait until catastrophe knocked at the door: bailiffs inquiring after unpaid bills; mother taken to mental hospital; the headmaster telling my parents I'd been expelled, and each of them telling him it wouldn't be convenient to have me back. No one very much did tell me what to do because they didn't know what they themselves ought to do for the best. And none of these dramatic moments, not even the things my mother dreaded, such as the neighbours finding out, turned out to be the end of the world, not even the end of my world, but were just a passage of chaos through which my life proceeded. It was erratic but still it went on. It was however also true, as the question suggested, that I was in general contrary-minded and had been for as long as I could remember. I almost certainly would not have done what I was told to do. My parents' track record in dealing with the world didn't encourage confidence. It seemed there was always another way through the drama, either by making a move or keeping very still and waiting to see what happened next.

After I was expelled from St Christopher's and on the loose in Letchworth for the weekend, I took the train to Banbury, to where my father and stepmother had moved from London just the week before. They hadn't bothered to let me know until the school stamped me 'return to sender'. I suppose they planned to tell me before school broke up, but my school holiday started unexpectedly early that summer. It also finished early, and even more unexpectedly, when on the Sunday evening a few hours after my arrival, my father told me that the next six years were going to be quite different from anything I'd assumed. Camden Council had given me a chance by sending me to a fee-paying progressive school, but instead of taking it, I'd chucked it away. He wouldn't allow me to go back to school at all, to do my O- and A-levels and then proceed to university. Instead the following morning I was to start earning my living in a job just like everyone else. He had arranged one for me. 'I've done some bad things in my time, my girl' – that's how he spoke: he believed it gave him a classiness that a boy born in Petticoat Lane could never hope for. He was also inclined to pronounce 'off' as 'orff' and 'cloth' as 'clawth'. 'I've done some bad things in my time, my girl, you only have to ask your mother, but I was never expelled from school.' During the recent war and after, my father had busied himself wheeling and dealing in the black market. He'd cooked at least one set of accounting books that had him in prison before I was old enough to remember, and somehow or other gone bankrupt more than once. Between the time when the black market came to an end and the moment he finally gave up his loftier aspirations and settled for Pam, the reliably adoring, tight-lipped, puritanical divorcee with a decent hairdressing business, whom I was told to call my stepmother (an inaccurate title since my mother refused to give my father a divorce), he made his living by lizarding around the bars of the fancier hotels to meet divorced or widowed women, and relieved them of various sums after charming the otherwise rational birds off their lonely trees. The daughter of a woman in Denmark had tracked him down and came banging on our door a few weeks after my father had left. She left much more quietly, having listened to my mother's tale of woe, and gave me ten shillings to buy a geometry set for school. So I did wonder that getting expelled from school stood so high in his comparative catalogue of 'bad things' he and I had done.

At the beginning of that term, the one I didn't get to the end of, I'd decided to operate on the bad side, join the midnight parties, hang out in town in a coffee bar of ill-repute (all the more dangerous with their glass cups and saucers containing frothy cappuccinos), and fall in love with a reporter for the local paper – a god to me. Now I had reached badness's logical conclusion: my schooldays at an end and a lifetime of getting up and going to work every morning. I was surprised, even shocked at this outcome, but life had been lurching around and about, my parents and I dancing an inelegant quadrille in which I ended up do-si-doing with him, with her, in this institution or that, and godknowswhere next. I'd arrived at the final destination, the actual godknowswhere I'd been warned I'd end up if I carried on the way I did. In my case, it turned out to be Banbury, above a hairdressing salon with a stylist called Rolf who put his middle-aged clientele's hair in firm rollers, and brushed it out and backcombed it into a warm fairy bun, and me off to work every morning in the High Street until I married or died, fitting feet into shoes in a supplicant position, kneeling, head bent, appropriate for one wishing to do penance. It wasn't at all as I'd imagined it, the godknowswhere I'd ended up in, but it certainly didn't hold out much promise of the bohemian writer's life I'd been hoping for. I'd arrived at where I'd end up much sooner than I'd expected, having had a swipe at far-less-badness than I'd assumed would be the entry fee. I'd been to a few midnight parties in the woods on the outskirts of Letchworth, the garden city of no one's dreams, drinking cheap cider and home-made spirits. I'd raided the chemistry lab and discovered that sniffing ether caused a most desirable oblivion. I'd been felt up by a few boys who probably didn't know my name, and had to face an angry policewoman who'd been called out when I was found not to be in my bed in the dorm or anywhere else anyone looked during a half-term when most pupils had gone home. She wanted the name of the man who had 'violated' me; since I was underage she'd make sure he went to prison. I didn't tell them that I'd been at the far corner of the school playing field with my beloved boyfriend, the reporter, fumbling but failing to achieve penetration even though he was on the trajectory of my dreams. Starting with reporting on a local paper, then national ones, and then leaving a salaried life behind to write the remarkable prose and poetry I hoped I could produce. But although I'd opted into the wild beatnik side, aped them, read all the required disenchanted books, talked the melancholy talk, wore big sweaters, black-and-white eye make-up and tight jeans, I never felt very much that I was part of the group. I was never comfortable, though it strikes me now that such alienation was the very key to the desired house of mirthlessness. So, after my embarrassingly short career as a bad girl, I was where I was, where women were notable for riding cock-horses and having no clothes on (or perhaps that was some other fine lady), and very little suggested that a bohemian life might be there for the having. I had some hope of a café that was disapproved of by the grown-ups, but events overtook me. I hadn't really understood how much my desired life depended on going to university. I sensed, at any rate, that a shoe shop in Banbury would not provide the soil in which a writer would blossom.

Doing as I was told, I began work as a trainee, paid £3 a week, £2 of which I was to give to Pam for my room and keep. Freeman, Hardy and Willis was a dreary, respectable high-street shoe store at which I imagined only someone without any interest in what happened below their ankles would shop. Someone like my step-mother, whose plain, Protestant hard-working life made me shiver for fear at its lack of any perceivable pleasure. I was at ground zero, the down escalator to the floor that lacked even a shard of light, the deepest dungeon with the blackest, thickest bars keeping in anyone with the slightest hope of something else, or even an insane fantasy that there existed floors above, through which one might glimpse a something more. I didn't take to it. My glamorous Jewish father (foreign, exotic) kept Pam (English, dutiful) adoring and fearful at the possibility of his loss, while his feet were firmly in the slippers she brought for him to wear while reading the *Telegraph*. Living in sin with my father was the single misstep Pam had taken in her blemish-free life. It seemed that being adored, and looked after, at this point in his life, was what my father wanted most, while all the desirable women, the well-heeled women, the beautiful strangers faded; none of them had lasted and I imagine that by fifty he just didn't have the energy left for the chase and the subterfuge. He saw that less glamorous women might offer the reliable devotion he now needed. He settled for Pam and all the excitement that she wouldn't bring him, the three square meals he could eat, the slippers she slipped on his feet every evening, as supplicant as I was in the shoe shop, and the incurious space and silence she offered while watching the television that allowed him hours of daydreaming about his lost opportunities and how easily they might have come off and brought him a life where daydreaming wasn't necessary.

Once when I visited him when I was living at Doris's, he picked up a paperback on the table beside his chair and waved it at me. It was *My Wicked, Wicked Ways*, the autobiography of Errol Flynn. 'There's nothing he's done that I haven't done in my time,' he told me. 'I had all that. Had money, beautiful women. I could have been Errol Flynn . . .' His words faded away as the reality of the patterned moquette he was sitting on reminded him of where he actually was and that patterned moquette was as good as he was going to get. On the other hand you could see that the heaven and hell of living in sin was as outlandish as Pam could imagine; leading a life that belonged on the left bank of the Seine tightened the muscles of her face and clamped her lips so fiercely that they quivered as if permanently on the verge of crying. But she had Jimmy and that was what mattered to her. Pam and I conducted mutual warfare from the moment we set eyes on each other.

I got on well with my fellow salesperson. She was ten years older than me, in her mid-twenties, and during the coffee breaks in the staffroom she told me about her life, the most remarkable aspect of it being that even after five years of marriage, her husband had never seen her naked. How was that possible? I gawped. 'Well, you keep the light off when we . . . you know.' And get dressed and undressed in the bathroom with the door locked. It was normal. Just as it was normal to be incapable of using words to describe the activity. 'When we . . . you know' was about as close as she got to 'fuck' or 'sex' or 'intercourse', and she was hopeless at describing the details of the general activity. This was annoying for me because I was so ignorant that I needed some specialised words to know what it was my friend was trying to explain, although I think now that there wasn't anything particular in her relationship to describe. I could say nothing about what was normal, since no one apart from my parents had seen me naked in my life, and one of the things I fretted about in my future was the idea that if I was ever to have sex, which I realised was a require-ment for a bohemian, how would I bear seeing someone seeing me without clothes? I had very little experience of sex, beyond fumbling in the long grass next to St Christopher's playing field, with all my outer clothes on. But even I found it hard to imagine an existence that required so much worry and attention to avoidance behaviour. A life behind locked bathroom doors, hurried changes of clothes, deliberately turning off lights when desire, if that was the word, struck. Separate beds, she'd said, and a life of taking great care to avoid the eye of the beloved. Not very beloved, at least in the way she spoke of her marital relationship. They 'did it', got it 'over with', and then led what my fellow sales-friend considered to be a proper married life; 'putting up with' and 'looking forward to', the latter mostly in relation to modern furniture, which had to be saved for. They went out occasionally with other couples, to the films or bowling. The marriage seemed unexceptional apart from the not seeing each other naked, and knowing as little as I did about grown-up living, perhaps that was how everyone lived. Her husband also popped in and out of the bathroom, with his pyjamas or his work suit, depending on the time of day. 'So you haven't seen him naked, either?' She screwed up the lower half of her face. 'Eww, no, thank you!'

All I really knew about marriage was what I saw when my parents were together. They went around our very small flat in all stages of dress and undress, in and out of the bath, with no concern about being seen naked. At weekends, I'd get into their bed and my mother would get up to make breakfast. She slept in the nude but put on a dressing gown on her way to the kitchen. When my father got up, he dressed in front of me at the foot of the bed. He turned his back to me, but bending down to get into his underpants and to fasten his sock suspenders, I was daily presented with a view of his balls and cock hanging, clamped beneath his buttocks, or sometimes, if he took a wider stance, swaying a little as he moved to button this, tie up that. I thought them unsightly, wrinkled and shrivelled, and his careless presentation of them to me was embarrassing, not because they were sexual parts, but because their ugliness was so at odds with his suave, polished exterior once he was ready to leave the flat. I didn't want to know that he had them under his trousers and white shorts, even though I couldn't see what else there was to be done with them other than hiding them from view. Odd that they were so present, but I'm unable to recall a single conversation between us about them and what they were for.

I usually air-dried after a bath. The flat was always warm with the communal central heating kept going in the basement by Bill, the boilerman, and often after a bath, in the living room, my parents would play a game of 'He', where 'He' was naked me, twisting out of their reach and running away from one, whose fingers tickled their way between my legs to my vulva, to the other, just a few feet across the room, gesturing at me, waiting impatiently to do the same thing. I bounced between them like a beach ball, squealing as they 'played' with me, all of us laughing at the huge joke of me being tickled and being unable to escape the grasp of one or other of my parents. The game stopped, of course, when my father left, first when I was about six and then probably some time before he left a second time and permanently, when I was eleven. My recollection of the game comes complete, straight out of the memory box. I see them. I see me. All of us laughing. Me shrieking. Being tickled is a kind of torture – it has its own page on Wikipedia. The laughter it causes teeters on the edge of frantic, with the apparent pleasure of the game and its acute discomfort as being tickled ascends towards agony. My running between them kept the game going. I didn't run in the other direction, out of the room, as I might have done. By the time I was exhausted with laughing and running, I was dry, and my mother would wrap me up in the bath towel to signal the end of the game. We all understood that such excitement couldn't go on too long, that I had to calm down and put my nightie on, ready for my bedtime story. One reason for keeping the game going by running between them was my being the centre of attention; another, stronger reason was that while the game continued and the laughter, mine and theirs, filled the air, the possibility of a happy family was sustained. Both my parents were engaged with each other, using me as a magnet between them. Surely that was a happy family. What we were like. The game was one of the very few occasions when all three of us were together, laughing, delighted; no one shouted, there was no crying or slamming the door, no one pulled open the kitchen drawer to find a knife, no one wailing at me about their ruined life, threatening to die. The adult me watches the three of us from a front-row seat, following the back and forth like a tennis game, listening to the high-pitched, breathless laughter. The adult me raises her eyebrows slightly, but makes no further comment.

So I listened to my new, experienced friend at Freeman, Hardy and Willis, who had never once been naked in front of her husband. One morning, sipping coffee, eating bourbon biscuits, she asked me about myself. I told her that my father had got me the job but that I had other plans for my life. At barely fifteen, I still had a notion of what I was going to do when I grew up. I was going to be a writer, I told her. She was impressed, almost as if I'd already achieved my goal just in the wanting of it. That must be very difficult, she said. I'd never thought of it being difficult to do, only that I wanted to do it, but couldn't imagine myself actually doing it, making it real. I wanted a job on a local newspaper and then – well, I didn't know how, but I really wanted to write.

My previous downfall had not been my last, as I'd thought; here was my next one. The manager had been passing the staffroom with its open door and me speaking of my life plans. He came in and said in stiff tones that he'd taken me on, young and inexperienced, in order to train me for a career in shoe-selling. I was sacked for wasting the opportunity he offered, one that other young people would give anything to have. Undeterred but rumbling thunderously, my father marched me to the High Street that afternoon and we went into the grocery shop, Cullens. I got the job as shelf-stacker.

I couldn't find any like-minded or friendly people to chat to at break time; they had their own group and I was too young. The boss didn't allow dawdling and daydreaming, two skills I did have under my belt. If he saw me idling (another of my talents) he'd call out and wave a pointing finger towards the shelves. Sometimes the shelves were full, but that was no excuse for wasting time, I should at least look as if I was working. My problem was right there. How I looked. It took only a couple of weeks before he summoned me to stand in front of him because he had something he wanted to say. I stood and waited while he gathered his authority. 'I'm going to have to let you go. No, it's not the work, or at any rate that's not what I'm sacking you for. It's your look.' What? 'Whenever I see you in the shop, you have a belligerent look on your face. I can't have the customers seeing that.' I pretended I didn't know what he meant, but I did. It was the look I could feel from inside my face, peering through the eyes, as if it were a mask which on the outside raised a barrier of contempt, a visible defence against everything the world could do to me. I can't do it now. It's a look that vanishes with maturity, like that thing you did with your eyes when you were a child, focusing them so that everything looked minute and far away but at the same time near enough to touch. I know I did it with the muscles around my eyes, but now it's gone. So too my belligerent look, which on the one hand kept me safe from all the real and imagined whacks (Melville's 'universal thump'?) coming my way, but on the other hand was so impenetrable that it made people furious and sometimes needing to hit out to break it down. That was the look that my boss called 'belligerent' and which made him want me out of his sight, and the look I gave my father when I told him I'd been sacked from my second job and shrugged in silence when he demanded to know what I'd done. He slapped my face. A bad thing, hitting children or even bolshy adolescents, but something I understood. An older friend, a million miles away from anything my father was, understanding, thoughtful, who gave me a place to sleep when I left the hospital for weekends, slapped me for 'the look on my face'. I can't bring myself to get self-righteous about it. I think it must have been terrible having someone look at them the way I did. Insolent, uncaring, challenging. And they'd snap. At the time, after telling my father I'd been sacked again, I really didn't know what my belligerent face looked like.

Sometimes I practised it in the mirror to see how it was to be facing it, but I could never get my face to feel right, to feel the way it felt when I did it naturally. It was perhaps like a spell, like a key fitting into a lock, it came to me, I did it, or it did it with me, and I was invincible, but stuck inside my expression.

It wasn't until I saw that look on someone else's face and felt the power it had over me that I understood how anyone could possibly sack a person rather than laughing at them for having a belligerent expression. From the inside, it feels as if your face is expressing the unfairness and arbitrariness of the world. You think that the look you have on your face is telling the world how bitterly misunderstood you are. How wronged. What injustice rains down from the grown-up with all their power? Although I could only imagine it as I went head to head with authority figures, the look on my face had taken in the unfairness and injustice, rolled it up into small balls with spiky edges and shot them through my eyes, killing dead the wrongdoer or the wrongdoer's representative.

I figured out that look when the alternative school for kids in trouble, which I helped run in my early twenties, went on a trip to the countryside. One girl of fourteen was wandering about looking blank hatred at anyone who came into her eyeshot. Everyone around was furious and getting more furious by the moment at the look of contempt they were receiving from her. One afternoon, someone had been shouting at her to say what was wrong because he'd had enough of her walking around like a harpy. It seemed as if others were ready to join in. I was pretty fed up with her, too, but on a hunch I went over and put my arms around her. In seconds she was sobbing and explaining what we all needed to hear about what was troubling her. It wasn't world-shattering, just something about how she felt we weren't including her in what was happening. I wondered whether that would have been the way in to me at my most silently belligerent moments. Maybe not a hug from the librarian, not quite the answer in the world of work, but in the matter of relationships it might be very handy. I must confess I put my arms around her with no emotion, I was still furious, and felt quite cold towards her; from my point of view the hugging was just something to stop her moody behaviour from ruining everyone's day. A few years back, I'd have dismissed it as 'phoney'. No real meaning or feeling, just appropriate actions for the situation. As mercenaries might behave, not morally on either side, simply doing what was needed to sort the situation out. Even the pretence of understanding and a touch with little feeling were enough to bring the girl back into the world of humans where she could talk and tell us what was happening. I saw that look in the reluctant girls I taught at an East End comprehensive school, and I saw it in my daughter and her friends. They could all slip on that superior air of belligerence they had at their disposal but not really under their control. It's like that very dubious 'multiple personality disorder', in which different people 'came out' according to what was needed to protect the central self, who had no control or memory of it happening. It's a doubtful diagnosis, but a useful metaphor for the withering look teenage girls can turn on. Try as I might, I can't recall any males producing it. Is it a girl thing? Does it come with a bottle of oestrogen? Anyway, that look was what got me sacked again and slapped when I put it on to tell my father what had happened.

I turned on my heels and left the room after he slapped me. I went up to my bedroom and packed some things in a duffel bag, found a capsule of speed (brown, torpedo-shaped, squishy) which I popped into my mouth for courage and moved the wages I'd been given in lieu of notice (all £3 of it, none for Pam) from the small brown envelope into my purse. Then I walked out, past the kitchen where my father and Pam sat with their backs to the door and out, away, off to try my luck in Hove with the other parent.

It was around this moment in the telling that my friend asked why I didn't do what I was told. One answer might have been that I had another place to go, and that I didn't *have* to stay with my father and take a turn at all the shops in High Street, Banbury before I arrived back at the godknowswhere which signalled where I'd end up. I had an alternative, a get-out-of-jail card: a ticket to Brighton to stay with my mother. But the bedsitting-room in which my mother and I lived for the next three days turned out to be more nearly the real where I'd end up, or at least the furthest I could imagine for myself.

The two of us shrieking, me saying I was going to go to London and find a place to live, her wailing: 'Yes, yes, go to London at your age, show me up, get yourself murdered and raped so they can all say it was my fault.' After two days of this, and seeing how hopeless my plan was, the small white pharmacy box with my mother's Nembutal really did look like the only move I had. Couldn't stay with my mother, didn't want to be with my father and Pam. Somebody telling me what I had to do would have been welcomed, and then, realisti-cally, dismissed by my mind, which by then was lost in a fog of choices, none of which fitted into the fairy tale or gothic horror we were acting out.

What I had going for me was teen rage, contempt impervious to offers of compromise; the power of the mask capable of turning ice to marshmallow, and all the time in the world, all the ability to sustain it without surrendering. In the cage-fight with my mother, which I knew would never end, just go from one ugly recrimination to another to another, a handful of Nembutal on the chest of drawers was the best weapon I could hope for.

After a stomach pump, and a few days in Brighton General, I arrived at the Lady Chichester Hospital, a refuge from both parents. A place as funny as it was sad, where I settled in with some relief to try and construct a future for myself. I applied for a job at Bourne and Hollingsworth. It had Soho no distance where the Beat poets and writers hung out, pay that was not turned over to Pam and a pound returned to me. No mother, no father (no Pam). Independence: the parallel universe where it was possible to get to the part of the world you wanted, instead of getting sacked from a shoe shop for wanting it.

I was to start at the end of March, but in February I got the letter from Doris offering a home. I sat on the edge of my bed, alone in the four-bed ward, and read it. And again. An entirely new world was on offer almost, the same one that had got me sacked from Freeman, Hardy and Willis. But I'd be already there, with the writers. And with just the single name: Doris (Lessing) she signed off.

You might think that after being offered such an opportunity, having experienced such unasked-for kindness from Doris and her son, been taken in sight unseen, given the chance to make real dreams of writing and the company of writers, the belligerent look on the girl's face would have vanished. It did. I took every opportunity to express my gratitude, promised Dr Watt, Doris and myself that I would repay the confidence shown in me and put an end to the sulky, angry girl who kicked against everything, especially herself. If my father allowed me to go back to school (the one point he'd set his face against, saying I'd have to show my quality and gratitude to Mrs Lessing for her kindness, by becoming the writer I said I wanted to be without the benefit of higher education – an act of jealousy that he said he wouldn't budge on, while offering only his gratitude to Doris and the promise of a pound a week which he would put into a Premium Bond account until my twenty-first birthday), I'd work hard and come away from university with a good degree and excellent prospects. All that. And I'd put away my belligerent face, which now, surely, was no longer needed. A proper middle-class teenage girl of her time, finished in ways her time extolled. Serious, studious, making Doris proud of me. Of course I would do all that and more to express my thanks.

But I was that girl whose face was twisted into a snarl when the wind blew in my direction and fixed it that way. I left school with a small handful of O-levels and no university education in prospect, made friends with the Covent Garden arty drug types, was living in a squat in Long Acre, and finally went into Ward 6 of the Maudsley Hospital. A friend of Doris's who came to visit me there told me that she (Doris) had washed her hands of me and expected that I would become a heroin addict, get pregnant and die an early death. I suppose there was a 50 per cent chance of each of those things happening to me. Or rather of doing those things to myself, compelled by my self-destructive nature, Doris would have said. The belligerent look barely had time to wash and brush up in readiness for hibernation when it rushed back to the face of its owner. You were very difficult, they tell me. You are very difficult, they say. It turned out that 'doing what I was told' was not so much following orders, it was some innate understanding of how the world was supposed to work and conforming to it, so as not to make trouble. By the time someone had to tell me what to do, it was already too late. 'Difficult' was how the lay population described what the psychiatrists called 'disturbed'. When all was said and done, I would be a disappointment to Doris as I settled in to the house in Charrington Street. She had made an offer of herself and her home, more difficult a thing to do for her than for most people, but in a very fundamental way, I wasn't really what she wanted. Imagine how frightening it must have been when, holding on to the new kitten, Doris stood behind the front door before opening it to me.

———

I was getting on as anyone of my age might, given my previous circumstances and the fact that I had been taken on, for I didn't know how long, as a house guest, or a foster child. Not all that well. I had lived with strangers before. I had been sent to a foster home while my mother had a catatonic breakdown and was in Friern Barnet, and later to a children's home, where we took walks in crocodile formation along a coastal pathway above the surf, as social services tried to sort my mother out with social security and a bedsitting-room, while getting me admitted to St Christopher's. After that, when I was twelve, an overzealous young rabbi – with Humbertian hankerings – sent me several times to stay with his parishioners during school holidays to help out my mother, and to enable him to visit me alone. He only shuffled on his knees across the room to ask if I would kiss him, and when I said 'no' never brought it up again except to ask if it had altered my feeling about 'our religion'. I assured him that it hadn't and could we please carry on driving to London.

By the time, two or three years later, that I got to Doris's I knew from experience how you tiptoed around a house that wasn't yours, fearing the sound of your own footfall, creaking doors or floorboards. I remembered not knowing the household arrangements, when was it OK or too late to get up, did I wait for others to have breakfast or get on with it myself? Was it OK to use this or that bathroom, which things were special to whom? I never knew the rules of each family or group, the systems, what is and isn't done in other people's houses and when. I always tried to make myself invisible and inaudible. Doing nothing was best, except that sometimes it turned out people were waiting for you to appear. I tried not to leave footprints, to erase any clues that might show where I had been and what I had done. But always eventually I had to decide to enter and leave rooms, to answer a phone or not, or to confront a closed door without knowing if it was the right time to open it. People weren't unkind, but I was never at home when not at home, which by the time I was twelve no longer existed, though it remained as a pattern, the only pattern of how to get through the day. It never seemed to coincide with other families' routines and expectations.

Once I stayed for a month with a strict orthodox family and after an intense Shabbos ritual of prayers, blessings and a meal, I woke in the night to have a pee and thoughtlessly turned on the hall light. The entire family ran screaming from their rooms, all demanding to know who the culprit was, sensitised even in their sleep to the grave insult to Yahweh that had emanated from their house, if not, it turned out, their blood. Towels and when to change sheets were always a problem. Toothpaste. How much water should you have in a bath? People had remarkably variable depths of bathwater. Everything generally was difficult. Using the loo during the day was fraught, having to flush and remind the house of my existence in it. If I were sharing a bedroom, I'd try and find some dark corner of the house to claim as my own, and I tried to keep incidental, accidental encounters with members of the family to a minimum, hovering on the stairs if I heard them moving about in the kitchen, returning swiftly to my room if they were coming in my direction. Which books could I take to read, how much loo paper should I use? Eating with them and going out together were all horrible anxiety traps. Their having me to stay was a charitable deed. A mitzvah. Nor was I subject to the natural forgiveness or generally non-lethal battles between family members. I didn't understand how rows faded away, leaving no one sulking. I knew though that I couldn't be a recipient of such forgiveness or such easy healing of wounds. I squeezed myself into invisibility, tightening every muscle in my body, terrified when there were arguments and small dramas that I might be dragged into them. Or I made myself known when I thought I needed to by a theatrically heavy footstep or a cough.

On another occasion, when my mother was stretchered off to Friern and I was sent I don't know where to stay with I don't know whom, I remember living briefly with some people who had a collection of coloured-glass figures – looking it up, I think Murano glass – and I dropped and smashed one that I picked up. I considered hiding the broken pieces, but the absence on the shelf would have been obvious. I owned up. It would have provoked catastrophe had it happened at my home with my mother. Here, everything was quieter. I could tell that what I'd broken was important, either loved or expensive. There was no hiding the dismay, but there was no shouting or screaming. I was told to be careful and not to touch things in future. I had no idea how to behave in such silent, sorrowful circumstances. When could I leave the room and get myself out of the way? What kind of apology should I make? Should I offer to pay for the piece? But I had no money. I found I didn't really like the neatness of controlled displeasure. Normally I would have clapped my hands over my ears and locked myself in the bathroom until things calmed down. But here things were calm even when I'd caused a catastrophe.

My first weeks at Doris's were like that. Having stayed in other people's homes before didn't help. (It still doesn't. I remain awkward and uncertain while staying in other people's houses.) It was worse, actually, because this wasn't a holiday and didn't have an end date, and there was no social worker or rabbi attached to oversee the placement, who could be contacted if there was a problem or my presence was too much of a burden. At Doris's house, I'd creep down from my top-floor room, past her closed door on the middle floor, to the kitchen for something to eat (did I eat too much?) or another coffee, knowing that no matter how carefully I avoided a creaking stair, or returned the cheese to the fridge, wrapped so it wasn't obvious that I'd eaten any of it, she would know I was there in the house. It wasn't just a sense of discomfort at being an interloper, I wanted to be invisible, not to be thought about on my own account. The idea I had was not to be a felt presence, to be a ghost, not to exist except for myself, until some signal said that Doris was ready to acknowledge me, and then I had to act my presence, shape up and be a good guest, however that was. But what signal? I'd have been grateful for a bell or a written timetable. I couldn't just ease my way into living there, or consider myself to be one of the party of two who would learn how to 'get used to one another'.

Doris had said clearly and often that I had the freedom of the house. I could eat or drink anything from the fridge and help myself to tea and coffee. I was to treat the place as home. (But hers or mine?) She got up early to work, I'd probably be asleep, but she didn't like to be interrupted, so I was to ignore her if I met her in the kitchen or on the stairs. (How do you ignore someone in their own house who has given you a home? And my mother had been in charge of etiquette. I knew I wasn't to ignore people. Speak up and always look people in the eye.) Still, if the door to her bedroom and study was closed, then she wasn't to be bothered. That was almost as good as a bell. She'd answer the phone and anything else that came up I should just use my common sense about. But I didn't think I had any common sense or none that told me when to override the usual rule of silence. Very occasionally a phone call was for me, and Doris would shout up or down from her landing. I'd rush to take it, excruciated at having *interrupted* her. We might meet over lunch and chat if she wasn't, you know, thinking, but how could I know? And she'd generally be around in the late afternoon and make supper in the evening. After supper we'd talk or watch some television (*The Wednesday Play*, *That Was The Week That Was*, news, documentaries, old movies) and then head off for the night to our rooms. I found myself freezing when I encountered her, as if trying to implode myself, and I couldn't stop myself saying 'thank you' and sometimes 'thank you very much for having me'. I picture myself in those weeks as traditionally Japanese: forever trying to make myself smaller, and out of the way, making my bow lower and my thanks outlast their acceptance. I asked what I could do around the house and Doris said, just the normal things. Keep your room tidy and help with the washing-up. My room was chaos and I didn't do the washing-up nearly enough. She was giving me an allowance and I should try to keep within it. I rarely did. There was, she said, no need for gratitude, that was silly. She offered the civilised justification: people had helped her at different difficult periods and one day I might be in a position to help someone else. I saw the mutuality of that and I hope I have in some ways, but it's never consciously been as a return payment to Doris. My need to express gratitude, the insufficiency I felt, was never assuaged by the long view. Gratitude was half of what I felt. The other half was fury and resentment, a leftover from all the chaos before, which in one way or another my parents were incapable of resolving. But also there was a substantial amount of anger at having to be grate-ful, the gratitude ever increasing, the bill never settled, and made more enraging by Doris's insistence that I wasn't to feel it. Also anger at the discomfort I felt trying to live invisibly in an unfamiliar house with someone I didn't know, at having to relax when I couldn't, at having to be at home when I wasn't. I didn't understand any of that until it began to come clear four years later, in another psychiatric hospital.

Doris's assurances that we'd get used to each other never cut through the surface of my discomfort. She had a way of offering emotional advice and making declarations of welcome in a distant, throwaway, clipped manner that expressed to me more than anything else her uneasiness with ease. The advice to relax came out like an instruction, similar in tone to telling me not to knock on her door if it was closed. She never seemed to be relaxed with me around. I began to get the impression that the words she spoke and how she actually felt were at odds. It was hard to know which I should attend to. Eventually I learned that they had to be kept separate, and I started to feel that I was in familiar territory, though not familiar in any relaxing sense. I'd come directly from a psychiatric unit, and before that I'd rebounded from father to mother, neither of whose places was anything like any home I'd experienced. It was as if Doris thought she only needed to say 'relax', 'don't feel grateful', 'feel at home', and it was done. It wasn't at all clear to me what feeling 'at home' meant within the context of the house rules that kept Doris from being interrupted and given that it wasn't actually my home. What kind of 'at home' was I to practise? Was I to be myself, the idle-teenager-with-a-bundle-of-anger-and-stored-problems 'at home'? Or a good-girl-brand-new-without-any-emotional-baggage 'at home'? The good girl was pretty submerged by then. I could, at best, remain silent and discover what practically I had to do or not do in order not to be a nuisance. So the first weeks went by. During that time I learned shorthand and typing on a part-time course to help me with the job at her friend's office, and, of course, because it was essential if I wanted to be a journalist, which was what I said I wanted to be to Doris – unable to admit my improbable fantasy of being a novelist to an everyday real writer tapping out short stories that became the collection *A Man and Two Women*, and writing the script for a TV version of *The Habit of Loving*.

A couple of weeks after I arrived Doris told me she'd made an appointment for me to see a gynaecologist. She gave me the time and address. I asked what it was for. To fit me for a Dutch cap, she said. The sooner the better. I asked what a Dutch cap was and Doris sighed before sitting us both down at the table to explain. I didn't want to get pregnant, did I? And it was really no problem using a cap, providing you took responsibility and never, ever had sex without first putting it in. But I hadn't got a boyfriend. Well, she didn't think that state of affairs would last long, and there was no harm in being ready. The last thing you need is to be pregnant and have to have an abortion. I tried to imagine having a boyfriend for whom I needed a diaphragm and how I would manage to put it inside me without his noticing. Being pregnant and abortion flew straight over my head and escaped through the kitchen window. I wondered if the predicted boyfriends were to be brought here to the house I was to make myself at home in, to be entertained sexually, or if I had to find someone with a place of their own.

There was an enormous amount of talk between Doris and her friends around the table, as well as in books and films I was reading and seeing, about the unsatisfactoriness of young people having to sneak about and use dark alleyways to have sex. Sex in dark alleyways and getting pregnant were pretty much one and the same thing. I wondered to myself how late I was allowed to be out, assuming I ever found any friends or knew anywhere to go. There were so many details I needed to know about how to live in this new world, none of which would have arisen with my own family, who had never mentioned the subject of boyfriends, but I never had the courage to ask Doris these very practical questions. Partly this was because I was a teenager with some odd questions to ask of someone whom I didn't know very well, but also because at any hint of a question about how I should behave, Doris would say everything would be all right and wave that arm dismissing my mostly unspoken queries, saying we'd get used to each other and we'd sort things out as and when problems came up.

This alarmed me. It seemed to mean that there had to be actual problems, clashes of expectation and behaviour, in order for me to understand what was wanted. I looked older than my age, and was a quick study. After a few weeks of silence, listening to people talk around the table, after a film, or about a book, I threw in a few acid or 'insightful' comments of my own. I turned from an 'enigmatic child', as someone called me, to a perfectly timed commentator on what and who went on around me. I acted sophisticated to fit in with these new people, who clearly valued it very highly. I could see I was doing it right. But bad girl though I was, and thought I needed to be if Doris and her friends were to accept me, I was terrified of anyone being angry with me, or of finding me out. I didn't know what would happen if I was found out, and especially by Doris, a stranger in whose house I was living. The awkward experiences I'd had staying with other suburban bourgeois families on a strictly temporary basis gave me very little idea of how to live as a familiar stranger in this house with Doris, who mocked suburban ways and values, and had such firm opinions about everything from politics and literature to sociology and psychology. And there was still no mention of how long I was to stay there and what would happen next.

I arrived at the gynaecologist's with time to spare. It was a private practice in a large house, heavily carpeted. I was taken up the stairs by the gynaecologist who had come down to collect me. She settled behind her desk and I sat in the chair opposite. What could she do for me? She wore a white coat and was, I think, in her forties. I said, as Doris told me to, that I had just arrived to live at Mrs Lessing's house and that she was a friend of one of her, the gynaecologist's, regular patients, and I had been sent to be fitted for a Dutch cap. Are you having an active sexual relationship? I said I wasn't, but it was for in case I did. The gynaecologist's face was a mask of professional inquiry. She drew a file towards her and took up her pen. She wanted my full name. Address. My age. Fifteen. She put the pen down and looked directly at me, as if I'd just walked into the room. What? Fifteen. Fifteen? And then she started to shout. How dare you come to me asking for contraception! You're underage. What is that woman doing sending you here? Doesn't she know it's against the law to have sex at your age, let alone for me to provide contraception? She'd be struck off. She was boiling and getting out of her chair.

I said that it was so I didn't get pregnant if I did have a sexual relationship. 'But you're fifteen!' she shouted. 'What are you doing preparing to have a sexual relationship at your age and then coming to me for help?' She moved around the desk towards me: 'Get out of here at once.' I bolted. She actually chased me out of the room, shouting still, and stood at the top of the carpeted staircase to make sure I left. I fled out of the front door and along the street, shaken and embarrassed. I'd come upon a world of professionals on the edge of madness, apparently. I couldn't understand how Doris didn't know that the gynae couldn't give me contraception. When I got back, still shaking, and with an adolescent's fear of the police being set on me, I told Doris what had happened. She clicked her tongue, irritated. It was too bad, X had been going to her for years and said she was very nice. I said that apparently I was too young to have contraception. Nonsense, Doris said. She wants you to get pregnant and have to have an abortion, does she? I'm sure there's someone else. I'll ask Z.

The urgency of my need for contraception was, for all Doris's explaining the catastrophe of getting pregnant and the terrible world of backstreet abortions, a bit theoretical, it seemed to me. A year before, living in Holland Park with my father, at the age of fourteen, I'd been raped.

I was neither dazzled nor drugged into sex when I was fourteen – I was embarrassed into it. I was walking along the street, one Friday morning, on my way to the Notting Hill Gate library, feeling cross after a row with my father, when a man with an American accent, in his twenties, suddenly appeared and started walking beside me. He asked my name. I ignored him. He repeated his question over and over again. That stuff happened. You just kept on walking when strange men spoke to you or exposed themselves. But this one was really persistent. He marched alongside me and then said that he was a singer and he'd written a new song. He wanted to know what I thought of it. When I said piss off, again, he started to sing. Loudly. These days, of course, I might well sing loudly in the street myself and not give a toss. But fourteen is different. I was excruciated. A man singing to me full-throatedly as I walked down the road made me publicly ridiculous and clearly everyone on the planet was turning their head to stare at me. And laughing. I was beside myself with embarrassment. That, at any rate, was what my fourteen was like. I hissed at him to stop and he said he would if I went to the recording studio where he worked and listened to him singing his song properly. It was just round the corner, a few minutes from where I lived. Then he started to sing again. He was amiable and quite funny, not frightening, if much too insistent.

I didn't think a recording studio would be silent and empty, I supposed that other people would be there, technicians, people just hanging around, but I think maybe I would have gone even if I'd known it was empty, just to shut him up. It was in a basement a block from where I lived. He unlocked the door and let me in, then he closed the door behind me and I heard the key turn in the lock. There really is a special sound of a key turning in a lock in an empty room. I asked to leave, and said I wanted to go home, suddenly scared, but he put the key in his back pocket and smiled. I want to go home, I told him, again, a little panicky. Not until we've had a good time, he said, and there's no point in screaming, it's a recording studio, the place is soundproofed. He pulled me by my upper arm further into the room.

Behind a glass wall there was that bank of recording equipment you see in pictures. In the main room, where we were, there were some mikes, a set of drums, a fridge and a sofa. I said that I was only fourteen and he laughed. No, I wasn't, he told me. I was, I said. He pushed me on to the sofa and I repeated that I was fourteen, and – I was pleading now, knowing I was in trouble – I was a virgin. I was at any rate young enough to think that telling him that would give him pause. No, I wasn't, I was not fourteen and I was certainly no virgin, he laughed, as he pushed up my skirt. I have no idea whether he believed what he was saying or not.

Even for those days, I didn't have much interest in sex, and I knew even less. I'd read some steamy books from the library, but the steam always obscured exactly what was going on. I really didn't know exactly what was going to happen. I knew it was sex and that I was being raped (I'd read about that), but the details were quite fuzzy. I was frightened, but not because I thought he was going to kill me or even physically hurt me. I was frightened because I was being pinned down. I was also embarrassed (again) at the nakedness of my lower body (I'd never been naked with a man before, apart from my father) and I think I remember even finding a space to worry about whether my knickers were clean.

The sex took what seemed to me an incredibly long time, much longer than I'd previously imagined it took to 'do it' from what I'd read and seen at the movies. I'd thought it would be just seconds and I couldn't understand why it was going on and on. It was also very painful – I hadn't known that happened either. Several times I screamed with the pain. I was crying throughout, and asking him to stop (I used the word 'please' a lot). I still wasn't scared for my life. He wasn't violent: he just carried on, refusing to stop, repeating that I was no virgin and paying no attention when I told him it hurt. He wasn't violent. I mean that he didn't hit me.

When he'd finished, he stood and straightened his clothes. I pulled down my skirt and sat up. He went to the fridge and got out a bottle of milk, offered it to me, and when I shook my head he drank most of the pint.

'You came a lot,' he said, approvingly.

I didn't know what he was talking about, I didn't know what 'coming' was. I didn't say anything.

'All that crying, you were having a good time.'

Apparently, my crying signalled a long and continuous orgasm to him. I wasn't inclined to tell him I hadn't enjoyed it – I didn't want to talk and I thought that contradicting him might anger him. I wanted to get out. When he'd finished the milk, he asked if I wanted to go for a coffee, but he let me go home when I said no, providing I gave him my phone number so we could meet up again. He must have told me his first name, but I have no recollection of it. Then I left and went the hundred yards or so to my house, where I went straight to my room, took off my pants and saw blood on them, and then went to bed.

I spent the rest of the afternoon in bed, sleeping a bit, feeling mostly sore inside and very blank. I was quite numbed by the experience, but I had also a strong sense of how stupid he was to have thought that I'd been enjoying myself – as I supposed 'coming' was. And I had a powerful after-image of him tipping back his head and drinking the milk from the bottle. Drinking milk has always made me vomit. My overall reaction solidified into contempt rather than shame. I didn't think that it was the most terrible thing that had ever happened to me. It was a very unpleasant experience, it hurt and I was trapped. But I had no sense that I was especially violated by the rape itself, not more than I would have been by any attack on my person and freedom. In 1961 it didn't go without saying that to be penetrated against one's will was a kind of spiritual murder. I was more disgusted by him than I was shamed or diminished. A different *zeitgeist*, luckily for me.

Nevertheless, for many years, I thought of the incident as 'when I got myself raped'. I was very aware of having gone voluntarily to the recording studio with him. And, that morning, I was angry with my father, who had just stopped me from going on the Aldermaston March. 'You can't go, you'll get raped,' he said. And the truth was that I was secretly meeting a boy from school to go on the march with him. He was bringing a sleeping bag. Once, in Trafalgar Square, he had, to my astonishment, put his tongue in my mouth. I hadn't thought we would have sex together on the march, but perhaps we would have. One other thing I remember thinking in the recording studio, aside from it hurts and it's taking such a long time, was: 'This'll show my father.'

My new friend, as I suspect he thought of himself, phoned a couple of days later and my father answered the phone, didn't like the sound of him and told him not to call me again. I hadn't told him about it, I never spoke of it to anyone until much later, and left the whole thing to be something that had happened. I did figure I was somewhat responsible. Indeed, an older, experienced male friend told me only a few years later that it was impossible to rape a woman: if penetration occurred she was willing. I hadn't told him about my rape, but

I wondered if I ought to stop thinking of it as rape, in that case, since I had been penetrated. I've changed my mind about that now, although I still don't think it was the worst experience of my life.

During my final term at St Christopher's I'd had a boyfriend who worked on the local paper and lived in Letchworth, but try as he might, it turned out I had seized up or something, because when we tried to have sex on the school playing field in the early hours of the morning, he couldn't get inside me. He'd been annoyed and said I was frigid. I didn't know the word. That, apart from moments and shadows as a child – the Humbertian rabbi, and the more or less unconscious behaviour of my parents towards me – had been the extent of my sexual experience until then. I hadn't the faintest desire, teenager and bad girl that I was, to know about or experience more sex at that point. Doris had made the assumption that a troubled teenage girl would inevitably be sexually active and therefore urgently in need of contraception. But Doris got on the phone and found another, more 'realistic' gynaecologist who, this time she checked, was prepared to fit me for a Dutch cap, 'as soon as possible'. The following week I picked up my prescription from the local chemist. When I got home I opened the box and found a pink plastic oyster shell, which I opened to find a brown and what seemed to me an astonishingly large rubber dome.

I don't remember the exact date when I went to live in Doris Lessing's house. I think of it as being just a few weeks after Sylvia Plath killed herself in early February 1963. The suicide was still very raw and much discussed by Doris's friends. So at the earliest towards the end of February. In any case it was before Easter, which fell in April that year, because at long last, released from my father's prohibitions, I went on the Aldermaston March. ('Ignorant, unwashed mob. You can't go, you'll be raped, and that's that.' Which was curiously whatever is the opposite of prescient.) I was quite heavily chaperoned by the responsible, twenty-five-year-old son of Doris's best friend, Joan Rodker. He kept a watchful eye on me against the CND hordes, and more particularly against one of his womanising friends who, not long after the march, would become the first boyfriend to test out the virginal, patiently waiting Dutch cap.

Doris hadn't liked Sylvia very much; after some friends who had been rerunning the details of her life and death had gone home one evening, she told me she thought Sylvia too 'pushy' ('networking' we'd call it now) and hadn't liked what she said were Sylvia's excessive overtures of friendship. She refused to join in the soul-searching and excited chatter about why the tragedy of Sylvia and her two children had come about. For the first time I heard that moral qualifier Doris used almost automatically and almost always for a man: 'Poor Ted'. Over the years the name changed, 'Poor Roger' (my first husband), 'Poor Peter' (her son), 'Poor Martin' (or any other man who she thought had been treated badly by a woman). But as far as I was concerned the death of Sylvia was before my time, if only by weeks, in the same way that the end of the Second World War was before my time at my birth in 1947. The two events marked seminal moments in my life, but, for all that I was surrounded by people intimately involved in both affairs, the suicide and the war felt less real to me than historical events that had taken place centuries earlier. I think it's a way of avoiding the intolerable fact that the world and the people in it got on, well or otherwise, in the years and days without my presence, as indeed, it and they will in my next and final absence.

It was a famously cold winter. I'd come from a snow-bound Hove, where I'd spent hours, sitting and brooding, wrapped up but shivering on the frozen pebbled beach staring out at an icy sea, writing poetry about seagulls and loneliness (no longer extant, thank heavens, though that's not to say that I wouldn't write about seagulls and loneliness like a lightning strike if I once let my guard down). London was cold, too. But Charrington Street was warm. Doris was particularly proud of the central heating, which had been bought, I imagine, with the proceeds of *The Golden Notebook*, published the year before. In the first week or two, friends came and sat around the kitchen table for lunch and supper, for me to meet and for them to meet me, Doris said. We went to movies, first to see Brando in *Mutiny on the Bounty* with Joan, who had been a staunch friend and fellow Communist Party member, and in whose house Doris had lived, and been looked after, for several years when she got to England with her small son. Writers, poets and theatre people came to supper: Alan Sillitoe and his wife, the poet Ruth Fainlight, Arnold Wesker and his wife Dusty. Naomi Mitchison. Ted Hughes, Christopher Logue (whose recording of poetry and jazz, *Red Bird*, I'd bought with my pocket money at St Christopher's), Lindsay Anderson, Fenella Fielding. A Portuguese couple, described to me as 'a poet in exile and his glamorous wife', would remain friends of Doris, about the only ones who did, until her death.

R. D. Laing was a guest a couple of times. I watched amazed as his wife (the first, I think) actually closed her eyes and dropped into sleep every time he started to speak.

I was thrilled to meet people whose work I'd read or heard of. I'd read all of Sillitoe and taken part in play-readings of Wesker's work at school. At Doris's I read Laing's *The Divided Self* and *The Self and Others*, and found a good deal in them that chimed with my experience of a mad nuclear-family life. I was aware of being on show, and was very cautious. I took the opportunity my novelty gave me to find out how to behave among these strangers. Doris made stews, boeuf stroganoff, salads, trifles, and we drank wine, Algerian red and Portuguese rosé. I sat, watched and listened. On one occasion, Doris took me to lunch with the Sillitoes, around whose table were some visiting Russian literary types, and Robert Graves. I was even more silent than usual, having a marked taste for older men, old men actually, and being quite overwhelmed by Graves's grey curls and the beauty of his pronounced Roman nose, as well as his grave pronouncements about art and life, none of which I remember. I was mortified that he failed to address a single word to me, although I would have stuttered into sawdust if he had. The following day, Alan told Doris that Graves had asked who that attractive young Russian girl was, and what a pity it was that she spoke no English.

For weeks I listened intently to the table talk, not daring to join the conversation, not having anything to say, and wondering where and how one acquired opinions, so many and that seemed to come so easily. We left cinemas and theatres, Doris and her friends and me tagging along, and before we were out in the street, they were sharing their judgements of what they'd seen. It was a matter of whether things 'worked', how exactly they had failed or succeeded. Nothing was expected to be perfect, so the conversation was about the way in which things worked and didn't and a judgement was made on the balance. Details of *mise en scène* and dialogue were picked out and weighed. On the other hand, Brando was preposterous as Fletcher Christian and wrecked whatever chance there was of it being a good film. How did they know such things? How did they make so many different angles relevant to their final analysis? And how were they so expert and so sure? We went several times in those early weeks to the beloved Academy Cinema off Oxford Street. Memorably, I saw *Les Enfants du Paradis* for the first of many viewings. Doris and her friends had already seen it, but rhapsodised for my benefit, picking out telling scenes or shots (*Vous êtes toute seule, madame?*), laughing at the way they'd been made to cry by such sentimental froth. But *Les Enfants* was too marvellous to be seriously criticised. It was certainly marvellous to me, and I listened to the talk after the viewing trying to find out why, along with *The Seventh Seal*, *Le Mépris*, Jean-Paul Belmondo and Jean Seberg, it was considered a marvel, and why Tony Richardson's *Tom Jones*, charming though it was, failed because it was self-indulgent. Self-indulgence was very often the reason for a film or play to fail in the eyes of Doris and her friends. It seemed to be a trap waiting for every maker of every art, and I couldn't understand how they didn't manage to avoid such an obvious pitfall, when it was so clear to the viewers. Although I relied heavily on others for instances of brilliance or ruination, surely the makers and artists knew what was good and what wasn't? Everything was talked about, judged, argued over. None of Doris's friends just went to the movies or the theatre for fun, however much they enjoyed it. Enjoyment wasn't enough. You needed to know how what you were seeing and hearing 'worked' or didn't, which sometimes was quite separate from how enjoyable it was. A film or a play was an event that only began with the experience of it. It was the basis for opinions, for conversations and for arguments that went on sometimes late into the night, over red wine, or occasionally a joint of the marijuana that, as an experiment, Doris had grown from seed in the garden the previous summer and which she dried in the airing cupboard with the towels.

Freud, Marx, Foucault, Canetti, Martin D'Arcy, Derrida, the anti-psychiatrists, even the behaviourism of Desmond Morris and Konrad Lorenz were to different extents the background to the chat for some, while others, Doris among them, relied on a belief in their own grasp of the effects of heart and mind on individual or crowd behaviour. But at that time, of all the ways of seeing in the world, understanding unconscious psychological motivation was everything, told you everything, i.e. the truth, while surfaces, behaviour, the overt story were so much gaudy wrapping – false reasoning, self-deceit.

I listened furiously, trying to take all this in and find out how it was done. To start with, I couldn't understand how it was so easy for them to have a point of view, to know how and why things 'worked'. 'Working', the pivotal valuation, was never defined. There seemed to be too much to learn. I picked up quickly that having opinions wasn't enough and that it was necessary to have a basis – from reading, from study, from hard conscious *thought* – from which the opinions were formed. But more important than all the theory, behind and beyond it, there was some ineffable *taste* or intuitive understanding implicitly agreed on by these talking, always talking, people. I couldn't imagine ever acquiring the all-important *taste*. Did you have it or not, from birth? Could you acquire it with diligent study? Many people were dismissed as stupid, especially academics, who apparently lacked good judgement, yet who seemed at least as learned as Doris and her friends. How could they be stupid? At fifteen, I felt it was already too late. I hadn't read enough, seen enough, been to enough places, talked to enough people. I felt that nothing of interest had happened to me, not understanding that every life is ordinary to its owner, that looking for interesting events was to search in the wrong direction for something that isn't absent because it isn't the point. I felt that I was burdened with a lifetime's weight of unfinished homework. I would never catch up. Never read enough. See all the movies and plays. Never learn how to think. These people all seemed so finished, so confident. And they *wrote* and were read, and by doing so they were deities to me, the hopeless unfledged writer whose sentences were never buoyed with confidence.

I stayed shtum. I listened. But I'd always been verbal. When I was researching for my book *Skating to Antarctica*, I visited an old couple in Tottenham Court Road who had lived in the flat next door to ours when I was a child. 'You never let anyone get the better of you,' she said. 'They were all older than you. You were only three but you kept up and answered back.' Already, when I was three. Protected. Armoured. Using words to get the better of bigger, older children. I learned soon enough around Doris's table the rudiments of conversation, even if I hadn't the faintest underlying faith in what I was saying. I knew I couldn't stay silent for too long, that silence wouldn't earn me a place round the table at which I was the only one who wasn't there thanks to their entertainment value, what they did or how they thought. I gradually stepped into the conversation, like the three-year-old keeping up with the bigger children. First with questions and queries, occasionally with comments and interventions. I set myself to learn, and asking questions didn't seem to annoy people. Listening carefully, I showed myself, offered myself to them as a young person who was eager and quick to learn. They were happy to teach me. So I learned to speak, rather than sing, for my supper. But I never, at any time, had any confidence in what I said or thought. Like a Calvinist, always already one of the elect or doomed, I couldn't think of myself as having that elusive and essential *taste* or understanding.

I recall two versions of me as I look back over the first few months of living with Doris. One conforms to a description in Doris's *Memoirs of a Survivor,* of how twelve-year-old Emily Cartwright settled in with the unnamed female narrator she'd been left with. The child is handed over and makes the narrator (in the film she was called 'D') extremely uneasy. The narrator interrogates her own feelings about this imposition: '[Emily] was watching me, carefully, closely: the thought came into my mind that this was the expert assessment of possibilities by a prisoner observing a new jailer.' Emily is described as having 'a bright impervious voice and smile', of being 'an enamelled presence'. The narrator looks for something in Emily that she might be able to like, but Emily always responds like 'a self-presenting little *madam*'. Mostly Emily keeps to herself, huddled in her bedroom with her creature, Hugo, a dog-like cat, or a cat-like dog. When she comes out she is immoderately polite, excessively grateful. The narrator recognises Emily's manner as an act, yet 'while I was really quite soft and ridiculous with pity for her, I was in a frenzy of irritation, because of my inability ever, even for a moment to get behind the guard she had set up'. Emily is indolent, unlike the industrious narrator, sitting for hours in a chair looking out of the window, while 'she entertained me with comment: this was a deliberate and measured offering; she had been known, it was clear, for her "amusing comments"'. Emily spears passers-by and neighbours with her acid insights and cruel stories. The narrator sees 'a sour little smile, as if she was thinking: I've got *you*, you can't escape me!' She almost enjoys listening to Emily's too accurate comments, 'but I was reluctant too, watching the knife being slipped in so neatly, so precisely, and again and again'. This narrator, who has other things to do, has been presented, for no obvious reason, with a damaged child, too clever by half, whom she accepts as her obligation, but struggles to like.

Memoirs of a Survivor was published eleven years after I began to live with Doris. She gave me a copy of the novel, as she did every one she wrote. It was inscribed 'To Jenny love Doris 25/11/74'. It made familiar and disturbing reading. I could see Emily in me, just as I could see my elderly neighbour's description of me aged three. It is as accurate a reading of me as Emily's harsh commentary on others. It is true, but it is, of course, a doubly edited version, a view of me from the narrator's point of view, which itself has been taken and worked for fiction's purpose from Doris's point of view. If there is pity in the narrator's response to Emily, it is strained for. I discovered after a while that Doris had a habit of describing people in fiction and in life as, for example, 'heartbreaking' in her most distant, coolest tone, as if to mitigate her dislike of them. She saw it as being fair, I think.

The other me I recall at that time is the me of my own feelings and behaviour, which seemed always at odds or out of true with Doris's analysis. The recollection of how I felt and behaved can't be taken as 'truer' than Doris's fictionalised me, even if I recognised what was missing in Doris's version of Emily. As she was described, Emily only got to express herself through the narrator's insights into her psyche. It was as if Doris didn't want to know, or it wasn't useful to her story to give Emily a voice or fears of her own. The narrator watches and analyses Emily's every move and thought, and while I recognised myself in those descriptions, I also remembered being quite opaque to her, simply because my recollection is of an interiority of my own. I put the two views together – fictionalised Emily, remembered Jenny – but they never fitted. Possibly that's because the bits of me have never fitted together as one is supposed to think they do.

In spite of my self-tutoring and edging towards joining in the conversation around Doris's table, for most of the time, we were on our own. A month or so after my arrival, I grew increasingly silent as I went about my life in the house. It wasn't just that early shyness that people assumed I felt or, as I thought of it, my watchfulness as I tried to gain a foothold where I'd landed. At first I was feeling guilt at being an arbitrary recipient of good fortune and at having left my friends behind in the hospital in Hove. Though it was to some extent adolescent dramatising, even sentimentality, I can't imagine how I could have got myself to think differently about it. But over time, a month or so, this gave way to something else.

I became increasingly silent in a way that was familiar and alarming. My mood plummeted as another thought came to me: a thought that hit me as if it was entirely new but which was perfectly formed as it dropped into place, as if, without my awareness, I had been thinking about it for decades. It was a realisation, and at the same time, a fact that I had resisted being conscious of until it made itself known to me, three months into my stay with Doris, with pinpoint clarity. It was a worry and a fear of such urgency and potential danger that it sealed my lips. I think it must have risen into my consciousness from a kernel of understanding that the strangeness of having been brought to live with a stranger was not just my situation and difficulty, but, if I stopped and thought about it, Doris's too. Somehow, it broke through my almost overwhelming teenage narcissism, and I did stop and think about it, and what it implied, until the anxiety became obsessive, and over those weeks I thought about it so much that everything else faded away in its shadow. And in that time it took on the form of a question that only I could ask and only Doris could answer.

As a small child I had regular episodes, which my parents called *moods*, and doctors would now diagnose as depression, in which I became locked away from the world outside my boundaries. I became mute and still. Not eating, not talking, submerged, incarcerated, unable to account for any of this to my baffled and cross parents. The barrier between me and the world, me and my parents shouting down at me, grew thicker and more impenetrable. I fell, was falling, deep in some pit, in darkness and alone, reaching a point of no return, when it would become impossible to claw my way back to normality. I sat in the middle of a catastrophe. I wanted to speak, though I don't know what it was I wanted to say, probably nothing specific, just anything that would break the tangle I'd tied myself and my parents up in. But I couldn't get the words out. Nor could I cry, so that he or she would understand at least that I was unhappy rather than wilfully stubborn and disobedient. Each demand to know what the matter was with me sent me falling deeper into the black. Each minute of silence, of 'refusing' to answer, made it more impossible to break through the caul I was wrapped in, and increased the fury of my parents. Sometimes the *mood* started from an event, some anger, theirs with me or with each other, or some resentment of mine. But often enough it wasn't triggered by anything that I could recall. Which was why I couldn't answer the questions. I didn't know. The only words I ever spoke were a mumbled 'Don't know' or 'Nothing', which fanned the impatience of my parents. These moods could go on for hours, even days. I can't recall how they stopped each time or why I couldn't make them stop at will, knowing that they'd stopped before. My childhood moodiness was no different in form or feeling from the depression I've experienced since my teenage years. I still become impenetrable for periods of time. When people ask, 'What's the matter?', the best I can say is 'Nothing'.

Now, at Doris's, with the weight of a terrible new question filling my mind, I fell into one of those black holes, and more or less stopped speaking. I managed polite 'thank you' or 'yes' and 'no', but I found it harder and harder to converse or explain. I felt I could hardly breathe for fear of what I was thinking. I was also terrified that my badness was revealing itself, actually creating the danger I was so anxious about.

There was a difference, though, in the origins of this mood. This time it wasn't because I was stuck with nothing to say: it was because I had just one thing I needed to say, the question I needed to have an answer to, and it couldn't be spoken. It threatened chaos. Better to keep it to myself. Yet kept to myself, it rendered me morose and silent and eaten alive. It was just a simple series of words but when the last word had been said, I feared it would explode and bring the house down around my and Doris's ears. It became all I could think about. Only one answer would make the situation safe. Any other would be catastrophic. But I'd realised that to speak the question, to ask for an answer, would open a door that was keeping my new world safely shut off from my old world. If I stayed silent, I was safe from the possibility of bringing the old world here. Then I realised that if I asked, and the door opened, I might not be able to trust the answer even if I was given the right one. It might be a lie and I would never know what the truth actually was. The black hole was the place that sucked me in, away from a world of double binds keeping me in the dark and completely alone. It was terrible, but safe. To ask the question was to pull the trigger.

I stayed mostly in my room and went downstairs only if I had to. I replied to anything Doris said in monosyllables, trying to be polite but failing. It went on like this for several weeks. Eventually, one evening, a Saturday, I think, after another silent supper which I hardly ate, when we were upstairs sitting on cushions on the carpet in Peter's room where the TV was, Doris told me to turn the sound down and asked me again what the matter was, why was I so silent, what was wrong? Her tone was kind and a bit desperate, and I wanted very much to relieve myself of the burden of my question. I wanted more than anything to dare to say what was on my mind, and to discover that it was all right: that there was nothing terrible about it and the danger was all in my mind. But to say it was to risk hell breaking loose. Hell had broken loose with some frequency in the threesome of my family. This time I was on my own. In a house with a woman who, in an act of charity, had taken me in without even meeting me. Finally, I spoke, and as I did so, I remember the relief I felt, how sure I was that once I'd finished asking the question, Doris's answer would render the chaos I feared a thing of the past, make my terror a delusion. She would make the question innocuous with a simple answer. It should have been a single sentence, but my memory now, as I try for an accurate recollection, is of excruciating hesitation, bursts of speech, as if the half-sentences layered over each other, a tower of Babel tottering as I tried to get to the right words and failed. Did I look at her as I spoke or did I look down? I don't know. These words. Something like this.

The thing is you hadn't met me when you wrote to me. It was incredibly kind of you . . . I'm really grateful . . . But now I'm here and you've known me . . . I mean – what if you don't like me? Now I'm here? What can you do, if . . . what if you don't want me now I'm here? Where could I go? You know my parents don't . . . I can't go to either of them . . . And I came from the hospital. I'm worried that you're lumbered with me. If you don't really like me, there's nowhere you could send me back to, is there?

I got it out in the end, after the rush and babble. The question finally spoke itself into the silence waiting for it.

And the silence remained. It continued for several moments. Long enough to start to frighten me. Then, still without saying a word, her face set and immobile as it had been while I spoke, Doris stood up from the cushion on the floor and walked out of the room. I heard her going downstairs and then after another moment the front door banged shut as she left the house. I stayed where I was for a little while. I had no idea what had happened. And yet in her departure and the uncaring slamming of the door, as I was regularly told not to do, I felt the ripples begin around my solar plexus of something familiar. It seemed impossible here in this place, and she so completely different from what I knew, to find the slightest similarity with anything I'd known before. In any case, I had no idea what had happened. Either familiar or incomprehensible, or both, I was terrified. Had she gone to the pub on the corner to get cigarettes? But she always had packets in the kitchen cupboard. It was dark, around nine o'clock. There were any number of reasons why she might have left the house. And none at all. Nothing that made sense of her silent exit into the night. Only catastrophe. The thing I had feared once I'd said what was worrying me. I turned the TV off, and went down to the kitchen. Her bag had gone. I wandered about for a bit in case she *had* just gone to get cigarettes and then I went to bed. I heard her return much later.

The next morning I woke and heard the typewriter clacking. I got up and went downstairs, past Doris's 'working do not disturb' closed door, to the kitchen. There was a sheet of paper on the table. A flimsy, like she used under carbon paper to make copies while she typed. It was a typewritten letter, not folded, the sentences more or less fitting the length of the foolscap sheet. At the top was my name, no 'Dear', just *Jenny* scrawled in Doris's almost indecipherable handwriting, and at the bottom another scribble, *Doris*. I read it standing up. It began by describing what had happened the previous evening. After weeks of sulking silence during which she had been increasingly worried and angry, I had finally deigned to speak. What I said had made her so angry she had to leave. She knew, she said, that I was used to living with melodrama and the psychological games my parents played. That wasn't my fault. I couldn't choose my parents, but if I was going to manage to become a grown-up rather than remain a manipulative infant, I had to learn not to behave as if I were still living in the psychologically poisoned atmosphere of my childhood. If we were to get on together in a reasonable way, like adults, so that I could stay in the house and go back to school to take my exams and make something of myself, I had to stop behaving as if everyone was like my hysterical parents. What I had done last night was unforgivable. She couldn't remember an instance of anyone trying to blackmail her emotionally as I had done. I was demanding and threatening, using the poor-little-girl-with-nowhere-to-go character to try to control her (Doris), as doubtless my mother had tried to control my father and me. She had never been so angry. She had been shaking with anger and had to get out of the house in order to calm down. She wanted me to think very carefully about last night and what kind of person I wanted to be. She was sorry if I was upset but it was very important to get things straight.

I learned later that she had gone to some friends and exploded with rage about my 'emotional blackmail'. The phrase wasn't one I'd heard before, but it was easy enough to work out what she meant. I had no idea that I had been blackmailing her. But Doris knew. I struggled with the gulf between my sense of my innocence and her knowledge of the world. I couldn't understand how I could have asked the question differently. Or why a question that was so urgent to me should not have been spoken, was wrong and manipulative. I thought that I'd needed an answer to my question. I wanted to know if she liked me, and what on earth could be done if she didn't. Now I saw clearly that it wasn't a question she could answer if her answer wasn't the one I wanted. The situation for both of us if she didn't like me was frightening, unlike any situation I had ever been in. My parents didn't like me, but that didn't matter, they hadn't chosen me. I should have realised that Doris was in a difficult position if she didn't like me. There, I supposed, the blackmail lay, in the speaking of the question that couldn't be answered if the answer was the wrong one. And yet it was still a problem to me; where could I go if she didn't want me after all? It seemed I was forcing her to say she liked me. But I didn't feel that was the truth of what had happened. I wondered now whether a positive answer could have satisfied me. Underlying the need to ask the question was my suspicion that she didn't like me much, and what I had done wrong was to be unable simply to live in silence with that reality.

I read and reread the letter. It was written with the icy calm of someone teaching an unruly pupil, seeming to give me one last chance. I was terrified. Perhaps it had been emotional blackmail. I didn't know. What I did know was that she hadn't answered my question.

And, though I didn't care to think about it in the midst of this crisis, what I also knew, and would know for the remaining fifty years during which I knew Doris, was that she had answered it.

After a few months, my father finally agreed with Doris that I could go back to school. I apologised to her for my grasping, embarrassing father. Doris laughed and said he was easy to handle. I had my doubts about settling back into the life of a schoolgirl, but I was ready to go to the local comprehensive after a full year of being out, since it seemed important to Doris. Also, I had to have a future – that was the whole point – and the only one that seemed thinkable in my new surroundings was to go to university, which meant taking my A-levels, which meant taking my O-levels. Doris too was adamant that I needed to take the O-levels I'd missed while expelled, and then the A-levels that would result in my fulfilling my potential. I had been saved to amount to something. I wasn't so sure I was up to it, but I tried to play along.

Doris said the local comprehensive wouldn't work, I was already 'older than the average thirty-year-old', and I needed somewhere that was more than a 'certification factory'. Her idea was that I should go to Dartington, another co-ed 'progressive' boarding school like St Christopher's. I apologised again for the money it would cost and which my father clearly wasn't prepared to pay. Doris, who didn't seem concerned about money until she was much older, said not to worry about that, she was OK at the moment, and that I might one day help someone else in some way. Her reasoning wasn't just liberal, it also tried to deal with the gratitude question I was finding it hard to come to terms with.

Her suggestion felt like a proper distribution of good fortune that took need and capacity rather than time as its fulcrum. It helped me more or less, by then situated in the dead centre of some new version of the rake's progress. In Tony Richardson's movie *Tom Jones*, which came out in 1963, there were waifs galore, dependent on and resenting the goodwill of strangers. But what could I be resentful about? Being resentful was the wickedest thing I could imagine, though it sometimes felt like a get-out clause for my guilt at being the recipient of charity, just a cobblestone's throw away from the paved pillows underneath the arches. Doris's almost arbitrary inter-vention in the life of someone who was already proving to be more troublesome than she had expected could also be spun into a useful truth if I could tease out the strands of gratitude and ingratitude and the reasons for them. The gratitude/ingratitude problem was always on my mind – it never really went away.

Dartington replied with a definite 'no' to Doris's long letter introducing me and explaining my situation, while keenly expressing their admiration for Doris's writings. They were sorry but I was too old and too long out of school to fit into their system and would be disruptive. (Later, when I was in the North Wing of St Pancras, I was sent to an experimental clinic for the young and depressed, but the clinic sent me back with a letter explaining that I was too disturbed and depressed for them to take me on. So my consultant put me on sleep therapy and every time I woke up, a nurse popped another barbiturate into my mouth, which I liked very much until my blood pressure dropped so low they had to stop. But that caused so much displeasure or panic in me that I tried to get out of St Pancras in my night-dress to find some more. The consultant sectioned me as a punishment, as I saw it, for their poisoning me, and several nurses held me down while a large syringe of Largactil was injected into me and I had hideous dreams and nightmares for days.) Doris received more letters like that one, and it was clear that no boarding school would take me, no matter how liberal-minded. Meanwhile, I continued to work at the office of a friend of Doris's who published newsletters about how to make the most out of the unprecedented boom in property prices.

The does she/doesn't she like me question (otherwise known as the emotional blackmail drama) was enough to keep me docile. Besides, where would I go if I definitively blew it? Stuck as we were, I knew well enough from my side of the front door that even in the oddest of situations there is a normal, no matter how odd to others, which life reverted to if you sat and waited, and though sitting and waiting has always been the least of my talents, it was the only thing to do, the question having been answered for me. The real events that disrupt the everyday, even sometimes cataclysmically, so that it seems that nothing can ever be the same again, erode, weather, change the underlying landscape, but no matter how transparent the platform you stand on, showing nothing but the void below, it hadn't yet actually broken and thrown me to the depths. There was a frost in the air. I learned never to ask Doris any question that could be deemed emotional. We continued with the business in hand: the upgrading of my overemotional tendencies, proving myself a good bet in the making something of myself.

This would be the point at which I describe the three years I lived at Doris's house as a schoolgirl from February or March 1963 until I left school and Doris's house two weeks before taking my A-levels sometime in May 1966. That is, a period you might think of as the early 1960s, although the 1960s didn't really announce themselves to us until 1967 ('Good heavens, so this is the 1960s we will hear so much about'). And then rapidly, almost concurrently, the 1960s started to be dismantled and we were soon wondering how that terrible woman telling us that there was no such thing as society came to be in charge. Or think of it simply as a time when my skirts got shorter, I often went barefoot around London, or hung out at home, which at that earlier point was chez Doris, acclimatising myself to her friends, writers and poets and a handful of people from her past political life, most of them rare visitors except for Joan Rodker, in whose flat Doris had lived with Peter, then four years old, while they organised demonstrations and international 'peace' meetings. If anyone asked later if she'd been a member of the Communist Party, Doris would give a deep sigh at having to tell it yet again, and explain she was never a party member. But from a 1956 article of hers in the *Reasoner*, an opposition paper within the party, it's clear that Doris was a member then, although she left soon afterwards. Doris unwrapped events with, I think, genuine conviction. One day at a party her then publisher asked where Joan was, and hadn't they been really good friends? Doris shrugged and said they had been useful to each other, but not really *friends*. There were several people there who knew how important Joan had been – looking after Peter and engaging with Doris's politics – and it came as a shock to them.

Even my semi-literate mother read, or partly read, *The Golden Notebook*, and asked me once when she came to visit whether I thought it was right, all that sort of thing. I thought she meant the sex, and the tampon moment that acknowledged that 50 per cent of the world menstruated. But when I asked what she meant, she said in a stage whisper, 'All that *communism*', in much the same way she said she was concerned about my being sent to St Christopher's. She read through the brochure, about responsibility and democracy, about giving children the right to have a say in the working of the school. She looked up at me and said: 'Do you think this is the right place for you, it's a bit peculiar.' When I asked what she meant, she said: 'They don't eat meat. And they feed you something called muesli.' Neither problem turned out to be a deal-breaker. I managed the vegetarianism and snuck in salami from the town when I was desperate for meat and managed to cope with the rather more-than-thrice-denied socialist tendencies of my rescuer, even though I don't doubt they left me deeply marked. Looking back at my mother's spoken anxieties, I feel a dim affection. At our best moments we had the makings of quite a good comedy duo.

Doris was still demonstrating with the left on international politics and raging about international matters, but I arrived at the time when, having left the party in 1956, she was still in search of something else. She was adrift, as she hadn't been before and wouldn't be again for a long time. She had had two serious affairs, with Clancy Sigal, an American writer who wasn't offering a stable masculine voice so much as searching at the edges of sanity with the likes of R. D. Laing. The other affair was with a psychiatrist from the Maudsley who, she said, had been the love of her life, but who was married and not prepared to leave his wife. When I arrived, there were a few one-night stands and weekends away with men she met, having instructed me who to phone if there was an emergency, but apart from inducting me into the secrets of good and bad sex during our kitchen table conversations, she seemed rather to have withdrawn or to be withdrawing from the idea of a settled relationship with a lover. Of course, I was there, and that, too, might have come into her invitation to live with her, either as a consequence or an excuse. The awkwardness of having me around as well as a strange man might not have been so accidental. No one ever stayed for breakfast, and when Peter was at home for the holidays an elaborate arrangement of a camp bed was erected last thing at night, so that it could be said that the interloper had missed the last train and had to sleep in the bathroom. I helped set the stage. She explained that a son should not be a witness to his mother's sex life. Six years later, at her fiftieth birthday party, she told me that she was not going to have sex any more. At her age it was demeaning to trail a younger man around, and there didn't seem to be any available and interesting older men. In any case, her interest in that sort of thing was over. She was still looking but not really for lovers. I can't say for sure, but it wouldn't surprise me if she did stop having a sex life at that time, and only later, under very different circumstances, did she seem to wake up briefly to her sexuality. Once, in her late sixties, she began a sentence to me: 'When I was . . . you know . . . a woman . . .'

In the early 1960s she was in search of people and books that would point her in the direction of a metaphysical education, an education for her soul rather than something satisfying her body. Around the time I turned up she was lacking a totalising commitment to materialism and an alternative to sex, which she began to speak of more in scorn than in terms of remembered pleasure.

The big love affairs were firmly fixed in the past. The party had come unstuck after Hungary and Doris was left without an authoritative voice, Big Brother or Big Lover, to give her a sense of direction, a map that would direct her towards a dignified goal. Perhaps that's part of the reason she chose to take up Peter's suggestion and allow me into her house.

The life she led was exactly how I imagined a writing life would be. She worked alone in her room and then she had a break, a social period. There were friends (some old friends, some fans, some writers from South Africa and Southern Rhodesia, and Americans and Canadians trying to get work in England after being blacklisted by the Un-American Activities Committee). She'd been accepted as a writer in London literary circles and shared a general forlorn hope in international social-ism, but there was no group working with some kind of leader or teacher towards something that involved more than her own personal development. In all the time I knew her, apart from that brief period, she had some sort of regular lover, teacher or leader. Then, having found Watkins, a bookshop in Cecil Court that special-ised in mysticism and occultism, she spoke to a woman who told her about Subud; she said that they were in hiatus awaiting the imminent arrival of a teacher from the East who was coming to teach a Westernised Islamic Sufism in a form modified to suit those who could learn how to learn, who could read beyond the words and sentences, and understand the intentions of Sufism. Doris went to her Subud group about once a week and waited patiently, telling those who were able to grasp it the truth behind what seemed to be slight tales and received wisdom. In the meantime she did yoga. She stood on her head for twenty minutes or so a day, and once a week did an hour of 'concentration' by fixing her gaze on a mandala. I was invited to the concentration sessions, which weren't to be called 'meditation' because that was what people much further along in 'the Work' did. She was only on the nursery slopes. I joined her on the sofa and sat staring at the mandala, letting thoughts come and go, trying to take no more notice of them than I would if a wind blew occasionally in my direction, and wished for some sign of progress, which was probably my undoing, because wishing and the Work were just about incompatible.

Instead of skulking about and hiding, I read like a hoover, sucked it all up. I also took myself off to the movies in the afternoon. The French Nouvelle Vague, the Italians, the Swedes. It was like a tour of the present time, with flickerings of the past. And in the meantime I worked at being useful in the office of Doris's friend, but turned out to be more of a liability, a maker of cumbersome mistakes rather than the Girl Friday it had been hoped I might be. Even if my father had refused to let me go back to school, I was having an education that was chaotic and fun, and listening to some of the makers of the wonders chattering over supper while never discussing their art.

I'd also found a different sort of gang of my own, from among those who'd been tasked with keeping me safe at that Aldermaston March I finally went on at Easter 1963, especially from the peacenik Lotharios who saw my tender youth in need of attention. 'Oh look at this sweet-natured virgin child,' one of them cried, offering his hand to help me down from the back of his Land Rover at the end of a hard day's marching to the not very urgent tune of peace and hope ('We Shall Overcome'). To which I replied with a cruel sneer, 'The fuck I am,' and jumped out of the vehicle unassisted, which had the effect, surprising to me, of sealing some kind of hopeless adoration for me to this very day. They were mostly youngish to middle-aged, though even the youngest had a good ten years on me, offcuts of the New Left who originally met up at the Partisan Coffee House, but were in reality, rather than political activists or academic theorists, more the hefty drinkers, convivialists, half-forgotten artists and writers, or never-to-be-known thinkers working their way looking forward but stepping backwards to oblivion. (It seems that elongated 'Some day-ay-ay-ay-ay' had the effect of putting off the battle for freedom and equality until they'd had a final drink, another hangover, one last fuck, or two.) I found these talkers and drinkers, ageing into a repetitive narrative and early death, very affecting. I wonder if I wasn't a cruel observer of those sad, flat-footed men, rather than a child hanging on to every vital word they offered me.

Nevertheless, they were the group I chose to be with in the evenings and at weekends, rather than my own generation, of whom there were plenty around. My older men were a disorderly group to hang out with, because finding them involved something of an Easter egg hunt. Actually they were rather more like slime mould, a species that has always enchanted me: myriads of minute individual organisms not exactly flora or fauna, nor quite fungal, that tend by some means, or some group consciousness they aren't at all conscious of, to flow or creep together in the same direction, so that they appear to be a singular thing on an intentional march towards or away from somewhere they had or hadn't been before. It would surprise us if we saw them with the naked eye as the individuals they really are, just as it would be a surprise to us to discover that our arms and legs were quite separate from the other bits of our bodies, yet through some unknown mechanism kept up with our torsos, or if you like, vice versa.

This group of the hard-drinking left flowed and tottered the length of Dean Street, and could be found finding each other by wandering solitary or in pairs in and out of pubs and clubs in Soho. First stop was the Highlander: you popped your head round the door, and if no one to your taste was there, the French Pub was next, just down the road. In the afternoons, when the pubs were closed by law to protect the livers of the land, it was over to the Kismet Club in a sleazy basement to check who was sitting on its foam benches trying to put enough money together to bet on a horse and buy everyone a drink (I put 2/6d on a horse called Just Jenny and it won a whole afternoon's drink for us). And there was the Colony Club, also in Dean Street, with the proprietor and model for Francis Bacon, Muriel Belcher, sitting behind the bar calling her favourites 'cunty' and those she disliked 'cunt'. I was too low on the scale to be called anything. On the slime mould principle, most of the people you wanted were usually to be found together in the same venue, talking loudly, smoking Disque Bleu and reckoning their chances with the women present, while the other places, often virtually empty, waited their turn. I was late to the party. Soho by then was not so much a resting place for poetic or painterly talent, but more of a merry-go-round of ageing drunks with and without a ruined talent, and just one or two with enough genius to know how to make their livers keep on working well enough for them until the end.

I should be describing the geriatric sex, the notable and scurrilous company, my often desultory couplings, my almost instant transformation from baby-of-the-bin to baby-of-the-pub, where my tough-girl edgy determination to find older, clever men who would teach me all they knew about politics, literature, art and sex usually ended up with me in bed insomniac, because the slightest sniff of alcohol meant a night-long vigil beside an old roué with little more to offer than the excitement of sleep apnoea, which required me to push or pull at the usually ample flesh to check if he was holding his breath such an inordinate time because of the breathing disorder, or because he was actually dead. None of them turned out to be dead. At least not when I was with them. As an experience, having a one-night stand with a man suffering from sleep apnoea was like playing Russian roulette, and given the physical condition of my aged braggadocios, as exciting as sex or conversation at the end of the hard-drinking day with them could have got. It was certainly a doubling back to my status as the know-it-all bad kid looking to make it up to her own Humbert (who had been, I believed on my first reading, so dismally wasted by Lolita), if I could only find him.

In any case, no one meeting me then would have thought I needed protection. There was drink, and there were drugs and careless sex (as if that were possible for a fifteen-year-old), and long discussions about politics. At lunchtime on Sundays, the fairground moved to the Tally Ho in Kentish Town, a pub that had live jazz bands, making it difficult for anyone to have a clue what was being said about the state of England with the vile Henry Brooke and Enoch Powell in the cabinet. If a trip into town wasn't to your hangover's liking, there was the warm suburban welcome of the Magdala in South End Green in Hampstead's lower depths, where Ruth Ellis had shot her lover (look, they've preserved the bullet holes in the brickwork outside) on Easter Sunday 1955, to become the last woman to be hanged in England. And that's how it was, all that, my rackety social life, the suppers round Doris's table with her engaged, debating friends, the one-night stands with lovers and leavers, the demonstrations against nuclear arms and apartheid, playing against a painted backdrop of what people would later call 'the 1960s'. Or just think short skirts, black-and-white eye make-up, pale lips and white boots with square toes and a cut-out rectangle in the front.

It's not very likely that I would have fared more freely and dangerously if I'd been living in the Bourne and Hollingsworth hostel (lights out at 11.30). But having moved in with Doris and taken the opportunities she offered me (the reading, the culture, the conversation), I felt like I was supposed to be doing this. Growing up, I would have called it. There was very little direction, as if Doris didn't quite know what to do with this unrelated fifteen-year-old living in her house. And I hadn't any idea what a fifteen-year-old was supposed to do in such circumstances. I only remember brisk notes on the scrubbed-wood kitchen table, telling me what I had done wrong, usually in the language of psychoanalysis. Mostly these were about not doing the washing-up, leaving my room looking like a tip and banging the front door when I went out. But there I was equipped with my Dutch cap and spermicidal jelly. More often than not sitting at the table listening to Doris – back after a weekend of peace and quiet to write, and back with tales of rapture in the shrubbery – telling me about her sex life: who was the worst fuck in London, who had been madly in love with her but was too dull. And I needed to know since the subject had been brought up why and how someone became the worst fuck in London. The answer was that the best fuck was considerate and kind, not in a rush, and definitely not one who fell asleep on top of you immediately after they had come. There was talk of anatomy. But time was the main thing. Time and anatomical accuracy. It wasn't only Doris: everyone talked about sex, in every possible detail. I sometimes thought I ought to be taking notes. The married bliss beneath the blankets recounted in full detail by one friend resolved my problem with my shoe-selling friend in Banbury, the singletons and their one-night adventures. The meaning of a certain look. The sex so overpowering that no words could be spoken, I'd know it when I saw it. I looked and sometimes I saw it, but being just sixteen (by then) I didn't have time to wait the livelong day for such a look. There was another look, more frequent, that led to the same result. The subheading of these kitchen conversations was always about being good or bad or indifferent in bed. I listened, and laughed along with Doris, but it was clear that I had to get cracking on practice.

But it wasn't really OK. Coming home at eleven o'clock with a man in tow usually meant a letter on the kitchen table, usually about noise, or, more often a silence, a withdrawal of comradely conversations. A friend of Doris's gave her advice. 'You must lay down rules,' she said. But it was the 1960s and Doris thought people of sixteen should know the rules. And as long as no one actually spoke to me and told me what the problem was I was at a loss. I wasn't having sex in dark alleyways, nearly always the cause of pregnancy in contemporary books and movies. I was being permissive, which was apparently some sort of feminist triumph. I said no when I didn't want to, and sometimes that worked. And above all, I was learning how to be a good fuck, which was what seemed to matter most.

As for Doris, her son was in boarding school, and she had been landed with me in her house. It wasn't what she'd planned. I think she thought Peter and I would come home for the school holidays, bring friends and a merry social life with troubled teenagers and lots of soup and wine, and then we'd all go back to school and give her another couple of months to write the next draft. But that wasn't how it happened. At least not outside the cover of a book.

All that would make a good enough chapter, Doris and her waif negotiating the permissiveness of the 1960s, just as, though entirely differently, the 'survivor' and her obligatory waif negotiated the post-apocalyptic world of passing hordes in *The Memoirs of a Survivor*. That chapter, the one I'm not writing at the moment, would start with an image to hang on to – and I will, I daresay, how could I not, come back to it – of the front door (black?) of the house in Charrington Street with me and my mother, dressed in our best, on the outside knocking to be let in; and with the wonders of the imagination that not even CGI can surpass, Doris seen standing on the inside of the closed door, with a tiny grey kitten (later to graduate to her proper name of Grey Cat) in one hand, while with her free hand she reached up to open the door and let in a nihilistic teenage life-form. 'She's your cat,' Doris said to me, offering it to me in her opened palm before we'd crossed the threshold. I took the kitten, who was clearly no happier at being part of this awkward moment than we were. Nevertheless, even before crossing the threshold, we had a waif each to take responsibility for, Doris and I. There was nothing for my mother, of course: there are limits to how many waifs one can gather together and fairly distribute as objects to care for at any given time. This was my given time.

Doris must have thought and discussed long and hard in preparing for this moment. Something new, a commitment, a link in the chain of caring for and finding a way to respond to something that was not one's own, not owned, but a responsibility to attend to. Or just a mewing accident that had shown up due to unfortunate circumstances (I believe I recall that Grey Kitten belonged to Sylvia Plath's children and couldn't be coped with in the aftermath of her suicide) at just the right time. Though for many years after that, all things that 'just showed up' at a given time were deemed by Doris to have reason and purpose if only one saw it with the right kind of clarity. They, the needy challenges placed before her as an obligation, young neurotic people, testy octogenarians, animals, plants, all had a role to be attended to, were put across your track for a reason. None of them (except perhaps the cats) actually loved, or even liked. Grey Cat bore no resemblance to Hugo the dog-like cat or cat-like dog that in *The Memoirs of a Survivor* Emily brought with her already set up as her obligation. But cats don't tell stories in the way that even the most respectful cat lover does. They do their own choosing as well as providing a simulacrum of loved and loving beings designated by the puppet masters of time and place. Grey Cat was kind enough to sleep in my bed when she was very little, and after that, almost as a gesture, had her first litter in the bottom of my cupboard among my shoes and grubby knickers, but from then on she was always Doris's cat. No one was in any doubt of that.

My particular difficulty is that I don't like writing narrative, the getting on with what happened next of a story that has a middle, an end and a beginning. You may have noticed. Sometimes the need to tell the story, to make sense of a narrative for the reader, feels like one of those devices for rolling up an emptying toothpaste tube, so all the paste will extrude and there's no waste. I'm much more interested in that closed door keeping people outside and in, separating and including. Or better, an invisible, perfectly transparent door to privileged readers, but solid as a drawbridge to those on either side of it who hesitate, knock, arrange kittens on their hands, smooth down their hair, find a face with the right expression, and then change it at the last minute, exhale, draw breath or hold it as the door opens (to them). I know I will have to come back to the larks and mess of the early 1960s, although, since I've written a whole book about how I spent them, you might do better to read that and then come back and see what happens when you add Doris, absent in that telling, as my grown-up in charge, to the equation. A kind of grow-your-own narrative. Just take some responsibility. But you are after truth. And truth, apparently, is all inside one person's head, not shredded and scattered about, to be ordered in any way you see fit. Was Grey Cat really grey? Were that lover's eyes so blue it was impossible to have him in my company for too long in case they clouded over and caused torrential floods?

I jumped out of my bedroom window so I wouldn't have to speak to anyone downstairs having breakfast. That's what happened around the Easter weekend of 1966. It was the last straw. For Doris, for me, for Doris's friends. A point of departure. My friend X from St Christopher's and I were still angry – three years after the event that St Chris had chucked me out without concerning itself about what happened to me. 'Well, you certainly fell on your feet,' the headmaster had said in a voice that told the whole world that it showed life was unfair but that Quakers would at least have the moral upper hand, and porridge. One for the Devil, but another chance to find someone worth redeeming. While I waited outside the head's office, his secretary finally lifted her eyes to show me what contempt she held me in and said: 'He's trying to work out what to do with you. Neither your mother nor your father wants you.' I knew immediately that she loved him and hated me because I had caused his busy day to become busier. My eyes saw everything from the time I was twelve until I was about twenty. They were faceted mirrors that told me exactly what I needed to know to understand a situation. So I managed to be rather sorry for her and her hapless love for a man who hated his job, had wanted to be a lawyer but instead had to carry on the family business of running an idealistic school for rich kids and a few needy children. Poor sod. He had told me that he was responsible for me as long as I was in the school, so after a moment I told him that I wouldn't have to be there if he'd let me spend the night with one of the day girls from Letchworth. I don't doubt this was nonsense, but he got me placed in the house of one of the girls from town and with a 'righty-o, see yar,' I swung my rucksack on my back and made a beeline for the wilds of Letchworth, where a party was going on. I belonged only to myself that weekend, and if I wanted to say something vicious to the secretary about not being wanted, I settled for a long look from my diamond eyes.

My eyes were made of diamonds, not the glitzy sort that sparkled and shone, but the implacably black kind that knew the worth of concealed things (some called them 'your coal-black eyes'). Those eyes radiated the truth of the matter to anyone who dared look at them. And the darkness drew in the world and showed me what the world could do and was doing. Those eyes picked out the lies, the faults, the vanity, the hypocrisy, and put them in their mirrored compartments and twisted them like a kaleidoscope, not into shards of chaos pretending to make sense, but into the actual truth, all unknitted and unravelled into what the fuck was wrong with everything. And what was wrong with everything was people and their need to do all those things that made the world go round. The answer of course was that everyone told lies. All kinds, big, small, monumental, trivial, world-shattering, mind-shattering, hateful, loving lies. No one tells the truth – that is the privilege of eighteen-year-olds. No one knew it, but there was the reason for the belligerence on my face. It was the visual representation of the fact that they'd never get one over on me again.

With Doris were her friends, a couple dressed for a country cottage weekend out of *Vogue*. X and I watched and saw it all. Sometimes we lay on our beds and laughed. Sometimes they appalled us. We knew that we would become them, and that was one of the reasons for jumping out of windows.

I had spent a week there alone with my friend who, having slept with someone as an act of kindness, had got pregnant. We were both terrified of what would happen. We forgot what day the bin men came, and forgot to dig a hole for the rubbish and we'd spent most of the day of Doris's arrival trying and failing to get a fire going for them when they got there sometime after ten at night. The fire persisted in going out. We gave up, cried and went to bed. We lived in London, we had no idea how to build and light a fire.

My window was a cottage window so it wasn't high enough to be a suicide window. It was more a matter of getting from A to B without anyone seeing my eyes, and what I thought of their complaints, when X was pregnant and the whole of her life was going to change, because I supposed that anyone seeing them and understanding the picture in the kaleidoscope would be broken up or down. Anyway, that was it for the grown-ups. We drove back to London in silence until we'd dropped Doris's friends and my friend home.

'When you've finished taking your A-levels, you will have to leave Charrington Street. You have been impossible. I can't have you in the house any more. You have been rude to my friends. You didn't make the beds or a fire for when we arrived. You will have to find somewhere to live. I will give you an allowance, but you can't live here any more.'

She said this as we were reaching the house. No letter on the kitchen table, typed and signed, no silence, no learning my lesson. Anyway I was nearly nineteen, why shouldn't I leave? I'd been impossible from the start. Asking questions that shouldn't have been asked, thinking they had an answer. I'd sulked: I don't remember about what, but I'm sure I did. I brought men home. I fucked men in Doris's house. I wasn't doing enough work at school (my new school) and for a while I had a boyfriend whose main wish was that I wore a uniform and who met me for a little fellatio before the school bell rang. I skipped lessons I thought didn't matter and sat in the coffee bar across from the school smoking and drinking coffee, reading or sometimes with a friend. I didn't work hard enough to fulfil my potential. I wasn't grateful to Doris for the opportunity she had given me. The woman who ran the coffee bar thought I was from the ballet school next door because I looked like a ballet dancer. I really didn't fit in with the fifteen- and sixteen-year-olds. I didn't fit in with anyone. Of course I had to leave. I was already bad. You behaved so badly, people kept, keep telling me. I look back and think: what if my daughter had behaved like that? Would that have ended in my telling her to leave? Who knows? The real point was that I wasn't part of the family, the kind of family which, my best friend explained to me once, always forgave you for whatever it was you had done. Instead of that, all the sulks, the temperament, the burning coal-black eyes. Once when I was in the bin (psychiatric not coal), Doris went to see my doctor. She came down to my ward. 'Doc Y says you're really ill because you haven't been able to take a family for granted. That you've been too good. But you weren't ever frightened of telling me any of your troubles, were you?' Doris waited for an answer. I began to laugh. I stopped laughing.

'OK,' I said in answer to Doris. It was time to go. What else was to be done? And for a week or two life at Charrington Street was straightforward enough. I found myself a bedsitter for after the end of A-levels and went to school, did revision. Everything was weirdly normal. I didn't tell anyone what she had said about my having to leave. And then one evening there was a phone call. We were watching TV, which was in the kitchen now. Doris's voice sounded low and doomed as she responded monosyllabically and then put the phone down. She said to turn off the TV. I turned off the TV. I remember an inward shaking with fear at nothing I could think of.

'Oh dear,' she said. 'Your father has died. Of a heart attack.' She spoke with great clarity so that I knew which word was coming next. I had a head-reeling thing, when you feel dizzy but it's the world going round at some speed rather than you going round the world.

'Oh,' I said.

'I'm very sorry. Oh dear, this is very bad.' It was bad, because a year before Doris had had me sign a solicitor's letter saying I wouldn't be seeing him again. And he had to keep away from me. This was after he'd taken me out to lunch, and given me an envelope, not to be opened until after our meeting, with a note saying he was going to commit suicide and listing my inheritance. Including his car, which I think he still owed money on. I had a bad couple of days and then phoned my father's house. He answered the call as if nothing had happened. This must surely have been emotional blackmail. I hadn't spent three years at Doris's for nothing. I became rather upset, another bad thing on our island of serenity, and then I signed the letter Doris put in front of me. 'It's the best thing to do. He can't keep upsetting you like this. You've got your A-levels next year.'

I went out to the local pub when I got the news. I didn't really know what a person should do when their father has died suddenly, and you'd refused to see him for a year. I had two whiskies. They didn't make me feel much better. Another place I didn't fit. When I went back to the house Doris came out of the kitchen to the hall and laid her hand on my shoulder. She patted it a little. Once when one of the cats had died she'd cried. She told me that her brother Harry had died too, but it was really the cat she was crying about. I tried to make the right words: different reactions, it was projection. There was too much to bear to remember. She dismissed me for banality. Which was right. She did mourn the cats more than her circle of people. So what? I'd learned that was possible too.

The patting on my shoulders with the front of her fingers couldn't really be called a hug, but she tried, and I felt strangely as if I should comfort her, for the effort she'd had to make.

'It's OK,' I said and went to bed.

A few days later, just before I hit the road to my father's funeral, dressed in white from head to toe, Doris said she thought I should be wearing a darker colour and not such a short skirt, but that I didn't have to leave after my A-levels. I could stay until I went to university. I said thank you, but it was OK, I'd got a bedsitting-room in South End Green and it was all fixed and I didn't think it mattered very much whether my father was alive or dead. In any case, though I didn't mention this to Doris, I'd told my headmistress two weeks before the exams that I was leaving school. When I thought about it, sitting on the playing field at King Alfred's, the day school that had agreed to take me for the past three years, I'd never heard of anyone going to university after school who didn't have anywhere to go in the holidays. Where would I live? It seemed an improbable thing and I certainly couldn't be bothered with the stress of three weeks or so taking exams. So I left. I packed my bags, said an amicable goodbye to Doris, thanked her very much and headed off to an attic room in South

End Green. (Eleven years later when I was breastfeeding my daughter, I mentioned it to Doris. I never had before. Do you remember when you told me to leave Charrington Street? Doris said it hadn't happened. She had no memory of that. She laughed with that laugh her all-knowing narrators have in her books and said: 'Oh well, if that's the way you want to remember it.' I'd seen her do that with people she'd written about in books, as well as people she'd dismissed from her life, but she'd never done it so directly to me.)

I imagined the relief of all concerned. I got a job in another shoe shop. I worked out that if I ate black pudding and boiled potatoes I'd be able to live on the generous allowance Doris was giving me (enough for black pudding, bus fares, silver spray to make my table silver). So I quit my second shoe shop and lay in bed reading *Anna Karenina* until the pubs opened and I went off to Dean Street to see what was going on. Nothing much. I spent all day and all night reading *Anna Karenina* and on Christmas Day, which I was invited to spend at Doris's, she found me doubled up in pain on my mattress, and made an emergency appointment with my doctor at the Tavistock. I arrived an hour late for it and bumped into my doc just as he had given up on me and was leaving. He took me back to his consulting room and asked me if I wanted to kill myself. I said no, I didn't have the energy. He picked up the phone, and evidently called Doris, his voice quaking with anger. How could she leave me alone in this state? What did she think she was doing? She was to get there immediately with a suitcase of my things and take me to St Pancras as an emergency admission. I told him that it wasn't Doris's fault. I just wanted to stay in bed. He said: 'Soon you'll feel as if you have enough energy to figure out how to kill yourself and do it.' No one, he said, could look at me and allow me to walk the streets in such a state.

Doris arrived, rather angry. She was given a list of things I needed and he sent us off to get them. Then Doris was to take them and me to the North Wing, the half of the hospital in St Pancras Way that was for benighted waifs and strays (remember *Briefing for a Descent into Hell*?). Ted, who arrived at North Wing with nothing of his past life, became my friend and we plotted to find a flat and live together. They put me in a ward with several demented old people, who believed, among other things, that firemen were scrambling up the ladders to rape them. Who knows? The sheets were wonderfully clean and ironed and I skipped into them, got out *Anna Karenina*, which I was halfway through a second time (although I loathed every character, especially the good ones), and told myself that at last I'd found the place for me. Doris left as soon as the nurse had finished filling in the forms. I was the baby-of-the-bin again.

Who was I to feel so angry? How ungrateful can a person be? Later I conceived the notion of teaching, and Doris supported that. I spent five years teaching interesting, disaffected kids. She kept in touch as if I was part of the family. Right at the end of *The Memoirs of a Survivor*, a novel as dystopian as any movie or novel now, She, the narrator, informs us that her clearing of an apartment between the walls of her house has revealed layer after layer of former inhabitants, and brought to light a 'bright green lawn under thunderous and glaring clouds and on the lawn, a giant black egg of pock-marked iron, but polished and glassy around which, and reflected in the black shine, stood Emily, Hugo, Gerald, her officer father, her large laughing gallant mother, and little Denis, the four-year-old criminal clinging to Gerald's hand.' Another mysterious She appears and is so beautiful the iron egg breaks at her gaze, and after some hesitation She walks into it along with Emily and her dog/cat-thing; finally Gerald, Emily's radical boyfriend who saves stray children, is dragged into the egg world by the children hanging on to his clothes. 'And they all followed quickly on after the others as the last wall dissolved.'

No, I don't know either, it was 1974. Pied pipers were everywhere, remaking a bad world. But I knew the cast of characters. Emily, me; Gerald, Roger, my boyfriend and free-school organiser with the children from the free school. The Survivors. Just a few. But what can you do with a benighted world? Only the ones who can see will see. It's a shame but you can't save everyone.

But actually, I didn't go into the egg. I knew my Humpty Dumpty and Pied Piper too well. Their survivors seem to do nothing but play Ring-a-ring o' Roses with garlands of flowers on their heads the livelong day. I made my play for a different kind of egg, acid, methedrine, dope, mescaline and all that, and finally got the egg out of my hair.

Four months passed in North Wing. I fell in love with Mr Amnesiac, and the son of an Edwardian poet fell in love with me before he died of the case of whisky under his bed. We played poker, and according to Doris, who told the tale in her own way, I wore fine grey tights but no knickers (I have no memory of animosity towards knickers, but it doesn't matter) and was sulky and annoying to the pitifully paid, hard-working nurses who couldn't afford half of the clothes I wore on their salary. But Mr Amnesiac regained his memory and fell back in love with his wife and liked his daughter, who was older than me, and reneged on our plan to live together. He went home, I stuck around and had a fantasy about a round room in which small people lived in the spaces between the walls. Eventually I left North Wing waiting for a bed to be available at the Maudsley. After nine months Dr Krampl Taylor considered me hopeless. 'She has a borderline personality disorder,' it said in my notes. Nothing will improve her, she will have a terrible life and lonely death. Well, words to that effect. I was young, attractive, wild, had my own thoughts which contradicted Dr Krampl Taylor, who also wrote in a paper that women should be in the home and kitchen, while men fought with giant mammoths to keep their feeble dependants alive at least for a while. 'You have an addictive personality,' he told me, and prescribed injections of methedrine twice a week while being challenged by the shrink so that abreaction occurred, and in the heat of the furnace of abreaction a new passive me would rise like a dragon out of the flame. The new woman. Made of fire and ice and everything nice. Fuck off, Dr KT, I said to myself, and broke into the drugs cupboard to steal more methedrine. Got on a bus, went to the Arts Lab in Long Acre, turned around in my chair in the café and asked the bloke behind me (who happened to be the speed king of London) where I might find some injectable speed.

There wasn't much sleeping done for a few days, then there was a comedown as bad as the worst depression I'd ever had. I left my best friend behind in the Maudsley and found other friends. I became part of a group. I belonged where I sat with my back against the wall watching all the words fly past me like a royal parade. Sentenced to sentences. I sat back and relaxed.

Well here I am at last. Comfy, with friends, not alone. Only I didn't know anyone's name, or who they were. But perhaps that didn't matter either.

That was when Doris crossed me off her Christmas list. Or thereabouts. Wild, dangerous, a woman with an active uterus that might do anything, and drugs as well. Hopeless. A terrible letdown. An experiment gone wrong. And not because I jumped out of the window, but because I had refused to take the opportunity given to me that millions of people would have given anything for. And I apologise to those millions of people in whose way I stood. If I'd known better I'd have stood at the back of the choosing room and let matters take their own course. No point in being sorry now. But I can see how irritating it must be. Sorry, people in your millions. I fucked up again. Gratitude. Not enough. Fail. So stand me on the headmaster's table at assembly to be shown up as the derelict I was while the head looked up my skirt (which he probably didn't, but it felt as if he did) and told the school I was the wickedest pupil ever known for biting that poor child's ankles when she had done nothing to deserve it. I am very ashamed of that. But I had my go-fuck-yourself face on so no one guessed that the most ashamed person in the room was me. Oh, but that was another time, another school. I was about six then and my friend, who was very small and I called Mouse, secretly took my hand, when the head said no one was to speak to me for two days, and squeezed it. My fuck-you face almost fell off, and I thought I might cry, but let it be recorded that I didn't cry. Not in any visible way at all. Horrible girl.

PART TWO

Chemo and Me

Tick. The final infusion of the three twenty-one-day cycles of chemo is done. I've been of a mind to follow Alan Bennett's excellent observation that he doesn't wish to be so familiar with the treatment as to call it by its nickname. But adding the 'therapy' each time has become peculiarly tedious and needlessly pointed. Back when, I used to pronounce R. D. Laing's name the way it's spelled, as he did. But everyone asked who I meant and then corrected me, 'Oh, you mean Lang,' so I gave up and called him Lang with a twang like everyone else for the simpler if less self-righteous life. So chemo's over.

A week after the last infusion, I was scanned from head to abdomen to see what, if anything, had happened. Just once the technician said 'brain' instead of 'head' and my careful poise unravelled, though not so far that it could be seen from the safety of her glass box. Maybe that brain-frazzled moment will show up on the scan as a bright spike in the terror region of my brain. The amygdala? The little almond, like the rusks called mandelbrot with their embedded almonds which I went on my child's scooter every Sunday to buy from Grodzinski's in Goodge Street. Next week, I see the Onc Doc and get the result of the scan, and the go-ahead or otherwise, for a month of daily radiotherapy at Addenbrooke's. Weekends off, just like a regular job.

So now I'm dawdling in one of those grossly extended weeks that one endures while waiting for lovers to phone or scans to be assessed. Why don't the lovers ring, and the doctors assess, the next day? Because: be reasonable.

You're not the only fish; not the only one with cancer. The world has its timetables and rhythms. It was precisely for weeks like this that our parents were supposed to have taught us to put aside childish notions of instant gratification for the more mature deferred sort. As we all know, come cancer scans and silent lovers, it doesn't work. So I'm living with Schrödinger's tumour. There it is: both smaller *and* bigger; spreading via the lymph nodes to the brain (or whoknowswhere) *and* halted in its tracks; in receipt of the good fortune (20–30 per cent) of a remission of unknown length, *and* the bad luck (70–80 per cent) of no remission. Until Onc Doc opens the box next week. I am interested in his opening gambit. The diagnosis came with 'What were you expecting from this appointment?' I imagine the opener to the scan results will be more of the 'Which do you want first? The good news or the bad news?' kind, because I'm beginning to get the idea that there aren't going to be any 'it's this or that' statements any longer. Superposition right up to the end, both more *and* less until the final opening of the final box, the upshot everyone faces, some having had more warning than others, sooner rather than later or later rather than sooner. Very few of us have an actual date even to pencil into our diaries, 'and so,' as Malone says, 'grow gently old down all the unchanging days, and die one day like any other day, only shorter'.

And what of the chemo? Some of the things everyone knows and dreads. Not all. Insane tiredness and chemo-brain, the latter not a Z-list superhero but an ugly fact of life as acuity and the capacity to hold anything in the mind for more than a moment drains away. 'You told me that, when? You did not. I'm the person round here who remembers everything. Remember? You did *not* tell me.' But when I had to ask the other day about a plot point in *Law and Order*, I knew it was my game that was up. Chemo-brain and tiredness like I've never . . . In spite of which I've tried to think myself into a state of meerkat alertness, to be, in this part of the memoir at least, a proper hack, close enough to the other side of treatment to report my findings on practical day-to-day living with an inoperable cancer diagnosis and the treatment for it. Answer: there is no practical day-to-day living with chemo and a certain uncertain prognosis. I gather that some people have chemo and go to work every day, undaunted. I am one of the daunted. The final infusion of poison last week came with an additional two units of someone else's blood to improve my low and unre-generated white blood cell count, and fix the anaemia that showed up in the blood tests they do so regularly. Iatrogenic disorders, but at least we know that the poison in there is killing something, the good along – it's to be hoped – with the bad and the ugly. So I spent seven hours – usually it's a couple of hours – attached to the cannula attached to a tube leading to bags of liquid hooked to the top of the chrome stand with a machine in its middle to regulate the drip, drip, drip.

Chemo-brain doesn't just dim my lights; it also has made me feel clumsy, not completely in control of my movements, as if the regular puppeteer is no longer the only one pulling the strings attached to my hands and feet. My superfast typing has many more errors, and I'm very wary of going down stairs or reaching for a glass. The main preoccupation, however, of the seven-hour infusion was knowing there was no way to avoid my drip-buddy and me going abroad for a trip to the loo. It looks easy on the telly, when the cancer patients roll their drip-stands along beside them as if they're taking them for a stroll, one arm outstretched to enclose the upright like an arm around an old friend's waist. It felt more problematic than that to me. Planning was required: any dancer will tell you that you should 'walk' through a movement in your mind, as well as stepping it out on the floor. I had to try to disregard the image of my contraption and me flat out, me hapless, the machine broken, and both of us dribbling pools of blood or escaped carboplatin (platinum, my precious toxin) from my cannula and its disconnected connecting tube. Think it through, instead: get down from the high-off-the-ground blue airplane chair; negotiate the bump at the threshold of the bathroom; manoeuvre it and me sidlingly in order to get the door shut.

Because I knew I would have to, there was hardly a moment of the seven hours when I didn't think about needing a pee, but I managed to restrict it in actuality to just the once. The occasions when as an adult I've had to give so much consideration to urinating have been few; most memorable was in the Swedish Arctic at forty degrees below freezing, failing to sleep in a tent pitched in a field containing 7,000 reindeer. I spent most of the night visualising the enormous difficulty of getting out of my sleeping bag, managing not to step on any of the four other people and one dog on my way out of the tent, struggling with the several layers of all-in-one and upper and lower clothing designed to make the peeing process a zip for men, but requiring me, without a distance-spraying organ, to expose practically all of myself to the herd of untroubled reindeer, while I murmured strong curses for their ears only, and my pee and lower body froze in the crazily cold, starry night. Eventually I just had to do it. It was neither dignified nor comfortable. But it was at least quite exciting and the sky certainly the starriest I'd ever seen. For the sixty-three days of chemo, even when not attached to a drip pole, my life has been largely made up of similarly lengthy considerations of mundane domestic and personal matters – get up, wash, dress, work, read a book, make a cup of tea, make a hot-water bottle, watch TV – and whether I can give a fuck about doing all, some or any of these things, or not-giving-a-fuck-withstanding, and going against every cell of my state of being, I should or could make the effort. The answer is, with the exception of the over-whelmingly desirable hot-water bottle, invariably no.

I was warned in advance about the cancer-and-chemo tiredness, the aetiology in both cases still essentially a mystery to medics, but for most people unavoidable. This I knew. I'd read diaries and seen TV and movies that dealt with this most feared and undesirable inter-vention. There is no treatment for the tiredness, as there is for the nausea, the other notorious side-effect that overtakes you. After a bad few days with nausea in the previous cycle, for the final infusion I took home four different kinds of anti-emetic, fine-tuned to take account of my earlier reactions. I don't even have to suffer the universal (I thought) mark of the canceree, her badge of baldness, because for some reason this kind or quan-tity or something of chemo had no interest in killing off my hair follicles. So I am grateful that chemo for me was not as devastating and disfiguring as it might have been; neither bald nor bescarfed, or throwing up, and thus signalling to friends and strangers which world I'm currently inhabiting, causing them in the other real world to shout across their sympathy and helplessness at me or scurry by in embarrassment. To strangers at least I'm just a regular stranger. That's something, or it would be if I went out anywhere apart from the oncol-ogy unit.

I listened to the Onc Doc's warning about tiredness at the original appointment, and wondered if he could imagine the extent to which I have always been indolent and agreeably attached to my sofa or bed. 'I have the metabolism of a sloth,' I explained. He said: 'This is different.' I thought: he thinks I'm exaggerating. Everyone thinks I'm exaggerating because they can't imagine contentedly spending a week or two – or three – not leaving the house, not once, and then finding it an insufferable intrusion to have to attend an appointment or even answer the phone. It's not a malaise, or if it is, it's my malaise and a condition I treasure. It's not a phobia, it's a choice. The Onc Doc and Onc Nurses talk about 'fatigue', not 'tiredness', as if to distinguish it in kind from feeling sleepy or lazy, just as major depression is distinct from 'a bit mis', or dehydrated is many steps along from thirsty or always carrying around a non-prescription bottle of water and taking a few sips from time to time. Fatigue isn't more tired than tiredness, it's differently tired. You can't feel the carboplatin as it travels through your veins, but you can feel fatigue in them later, as though they were filled with sluggish liquidised metal (mercury, say, but without the 'quick' of quicksilver) dragging its weighty way around your body, to your arms, legs, head, fingers, torso, and to eyelids that feel so heavy they threaten to drain down into a viscous puddle at your feet, your veins imploded and sucked dry by a monstrous gravity. Anyway, very tired Fatigue.

A regular day now might unfold with me doing some work in bed and then getting up. Showering or bathing and dressing, and then, all clean and ready for the day, the body and mind refold themselves, suddenly faced with the urgent decision whether to eat something or to get back into bed straight away, not stopping for food, to sleep for four more hours or so. With or without breakfast, the effort of getting up finishes the day off for me. I've tried it the other way round, getting up first, before work, but then that's as far as I get, so no breakfast and no work, peeling off the clothes I've just put on and creeping back to bed, with nothing done, but mightily relieved to have been let off the exhausting business of making a decision. Logically, I should stay in bed all day and work intermittently, like snacking, as well as snacking intermittently, like snacking. But my brain and muscles turn off after a while of working, so I'd have to go back to sleep again, anyway, not dozing, no forty winks, but deeply, fast, vastly asleep. And as the Macmillan Nurse booklets (every patient's and, it seems, every doctor's source of information) explain, this fatigue is not alleviated by rest. You wake up just as exhausted as you were when you went to sleep. In an aside, they say that the fatigue can last between two months and two years *after* the chemo has finished. In a few months (or years) of days like that, a full consideration of the necessity or otherwise of having a pee counts as quite exciting enough. I've tried but failed to watch a full-length episode of *Lovejoy*, the Poet's favourite after a day wording and teaching, but my lowered excitement threshold can't take the plot tensions or the anguish of seeing those familiar youthful faces of now-aged English actors who you just can't put a name to, though it's on the tip of your tongue. That's how fatigued I've been. After the blood transfusion, I'd hoped for something like Popeye's transfiguration after downing a tin of spinach, but I was still pretty tired in the days after. I could sleep in a heartbeat, but my veins were filled with something lighter than mercury, and my body was not so determined to join in with my mind's unchanged exhaustion. It was an improvement, but by Day 6 the full weight of exhaustion – had the new blood run out? – hit me like a wrecking ball and I spent that weekend asleep for ten and more hours of daytime after eight or nine hours at night.

Days, by the way, are my new way of telling time. They are the units of chemo, Day 1 to Day 21, after which it all starts again at Day 1. Day 6 or 7 is the lowest ebb and in each cycle, I have to start a course of antibiotics to fend off infection. I'm supposed to pick up by Day 15 or 16, my blood recovering, but I've never noticed it, and the need for the blood transfusion last time suggests that my body isn't playing strictly to the prescribed rhythm. The body, we shouldn't be surprised to learn, has a mind of its own.

The chemo period, for all the deadness of feeling and lack of fine-tuning, threw a lasso round my life. Until the three cycles were complete, nothing else was going to happen. There was stasis in the other, non-cancer life. Not just exhaustion, but a lack of will even to investigate what was going on inside me. I feel I've allowed myself more ignorance about the nature and behaviour of my cancer than I'd allow myself if I had the flu. I am not a doctor, but there's the Internet and I'm still capable of reading, if not retaining, say, a juicy paper at Academia.edu: 'Things Fall Apart: Heidegger on the Constancy and Finality of Death' (by Taylor Carman), so how come I've remained so foggy about the details and possible trajectories of my cancer? I tell myself it's because I'm not so much in charge in cancer-world. I don't think I've ever felt so not in charge. This is one of the surprises of being cancered. I don't approve, but I don't have the energy to roll up my sleeves and find out everything there is to be found. The exhaustion makes me incapable, but there is also some absence of will to find everything out. On the other hand, it's also increasingly clear to me that there may be little to find out and that no one, Onc Doc, Onc Nurse, really knows very much, except in an academic way. Everything is presented to me statistically, as probabilities. I can't find the right question to break through that, to talk about the cancer that is me and mine, what it is, how it is, how it and I are with each other. Something that pans in on the singularity of the particular cancer I'm hosting. I guess it's because 'they don't know', like they don't know exactly how or why antidepressants work, but that they do, statistically well enough.

I think, all they can do with me and my cancer is to follow the cancer's lead. The scan will show if the tumour has shrunk or stayed still, it will show where it has travelled to, 'except', Onc Doc explains, 'where it's too small for us to see'. This crucial exception means waiting for it to grow (get worse) to know where and how far it has gone, when it will also have moved on to be invisibly small somewhere else. The Red Queen explains it in *Looking-Glass* world: 'Now *here,* you see, it takes all the running you can do, to keep in the same place.' *Looking-Glass* world is more stressful in this respect than *Wonderland*, my preferred state of being, where participants in the Caucus-race start to run when they like and leave off when they like and 'everybody has won, and all must have prizes'. In moments of crisis the Alice books have always offered me the common sense of my situation. They are whispering in my ear incessantly in my cancer life.

The treatment seems to be not so very different from what it was decades ago. A plug-ugly poison that kills off cancer cells faster than it kills off other cells. They think. Then checking to see if it has done anything useful. Maybe it has, maybe it hasn't. Everyone is waiting to see what is going to happen in order to know what is going to happen. The cancer's in charge and leading them all a merry dance. Perhaps that's why I've so little taste for investigation. There's an awful lot of uncertainty for patients and doctors in this cancer business. And uncertainty is what I am least good at. I've always been prepared to use extreme measures, find drastic solutions, to put an end to uncertainty in my life. (We are back at my failed training in deferred gratification.) As far as I can see this cancer thing has left me without any measures to use or solutions to find. My sense of being a patient, with all its unwelcome connotations, is inescapable. I might refuse treatment, to which, already, Onc Doc has nodded and said that, yes, that is one path open to me which he would respect. So dumb refusal, too, is incorporated into this world. There is no way to be an impatient, or a mispatient, or even an unruly patient. Cancer-world is so structured that one has to proceed as if one were a grown-up, with all its unwelcome connotations.

What has most surprised me is that as soon as I arrived at the oncology day ward for the final infusion, I found myself anxious, distressed even, that there would be no more visits to the ward. I worried that 'my' designated nurse, L, would no longer be available to be called, as she insists, with 'any little problem, no matter how small'. The kindness of nurses is remarkable. The mystery is not that some are said to be heartless, to have had their fill of sick, moaning patients and claptrap bureaucracy, but that so few are like that. Your anonymity to them – you're not their pal or their sister – makes their patience and friendliness all the more astonishing and truly valuable if you are sick or frightened. So, hampered as I am at rebellion, I've now discovered myself to be a little attached to Nurse L's unfailing availability and good humour. In fact I was already, in advance, missing the whole thing: the trips to the ward itself; the reception, and G, the always smiling, carefully dressed receptionist; Schindler's lift, the world's slowest elevator, with life-saving equipment on the wall in case it failed to get you there in time; the ghastly brown autumnal prints on the corridor walls; and even, in a distant way, the other patients. We hardly spoke to one another, but only nodded our heads, because people in various stages of cancer treatment aren't a group anyone wants to be a part of. My former mother-in-law went to the Bristol centre for alternative cancer therapy and in between juicing fields-worth of carrots, complained until her own death about the letters she regularly received from spouses, informing her that one of their group had died. She said it wasn't encouraging.

The oncology day ward exists solely for people who are anxious and sick, and their frightened relatives, and is staffed by people trained to deal with those conditions. You might think, I did think, it would be a relief to shake the carpet static from my shoes. Yet, on my last day, I discovered that there was something about the entire, dreaded, much mythologised and allegorised cancer ward and its inhabitants, perhaps the pathos, that attaches you to it, however delicate or elastic the connecting fibre. It took me a few minutes to recognise what I was feeling. Over a couple of months of, as I thought, carefully observed treatment, I'd already become mildly institutionalised. Even while I sat there being infused, I felt the loss of the unlovely place and the nurses who, however kind they might be, you rationally hoped you wouldn't be seeing again soon. So much for my cold eye on life, on death. I have the feeling of being sent away from a place of safety. Left outside. *Peter Pan – Peter Panic*: not just the awfully big adventure, also the tap-tap-tapping on the window to be let back in. And I'm further along the programme, a step nearer the end. Where are the place and people I can turn to now – the 'designated' nurse I can call my own? Will there be a person there for me if and when I start the radiation therapy, or will I just go to the room where the machine is housed (its technicians sit in another room to avoid the rays) and be zapped day by day for a month, then wait for another scan, another assessment from the Onc Doc, without having someone on the end of a telephone for 'any little problem, no matter how small'? What am I, ten years old? At best, I think, at the moment.

That institutionalisation and the inner seethings of loss, I remember well enough from leaving schools both as a pupil and as a teacher, and my stays, long ago, in psychiatric units; the tug, the claim, that such places and the people in them have on your emotions, the falling away of the safety net and the fearful feeling of privation when your time as part of a system runs out. In Hove, during my first hospitalisation at fifteen, in the small unit where they kept a kindly eye on me, both staff and patients, I'd felt such resistance and fear the day I left with my mother to go and live with Doris. I had three or four particular friends, all strikingly different from one another and from me, but closely woven together as inmates. They expressed real pleasure at my 'fairy-tale ending', no resentment that it wasn't them being taken away to some glamorous London life and being wanted, sight unseen, by somebody. Anyway, one of them said, 'If it can happen to you it can happen to us,' so with the generosity of inmates, they allowed me to represent possibility for them. Leaving them was a wrench. Leaving them behind filled me with a sense of unfairness, which, not much later, when I was reading accounts of the Holocaust, I recognised as a minor form of survivor guilt.

They wrote to me in London and gave me the gossip, which was normal for life in the Lady Chichester, but hilarious, wilder and more poignant than most everyday goings-on. Pam, after sitting in a cold bath to shrink her Levi's in the approved way, had a panic attack, and had to be cut out of her saturated skintight jeans; Sally hadn't left her bed for a week and Dr Watt was threatening her with the one-way ticket to Haywards Heath, the big asylum that everyone knew no one returned from; Stuart had done a drawing of a sporran in art therapy, claiming his Scottish origins, he said, but his psychiatrist had shaken his head and looked intently at him. 'A sporran, you say, a sporran? And what is behind a sporran?' Stuart, who was famously excruciated at the thought of anything physical, said, 'A kilt,' but his shrink wasn't having it. 'And what is behind the kilt, Stuart?' Stuart finally fessed up to owning a penis and had to be put on stronger tranquillisers for a few days. This last story was told in great confidence to Margaret, who said that she didn't think the confidentiality applied to me as I was no longer part of daily life at the Lady C. Everyone sent their love and, although none of them was a reader or had heard of her, they were eager to know how I, the wannabe writer who had escaped the bin, was getting on in the house of the famous novelist.

———

The treatment's over and done with. First from August to October, the three cycles of chemotherapy, then I graduated from the poison infusions to the death rays, with daily radiotherapy. When I look back from my current spot in the land of hiatus, the entire process makes me think of clubbing baby seals, although the seals I'm familiar with aren't adorable chubby babies, but glossy, black, athletic adults leaping for fish at feeding time in London Zoo when I was small, and gigantic elephant seals lounging on the shore in an Antarctic bay, paying not the slightest attention to me as I picked my way through the spaces they leave between them. Vast blubber sacks, lolling, shapeless with fat, their truncated trunks flaccid, concealing lipstick-red mouths and throats that appear when they open wide to yawn. No, not them: baby seals, small, helpless, newborn, cute, white ones with big watery eyes. This probably isn't the right attitude to cancer treatment. I'm feeling oppressed.

I grew grumpy, at best, during my daily encounters with the machine I learned was called an Elekta Linear Accelerator, and those who attended it. The radiographers were all young, mostly in their twenties or early thirties. Two of them were amiable, but I only saw them three times; the rest were more interested in getting my body to conform to the co-ordinates set at the first planning visit than in noticing there was a person attached to the flesh they pushed and pulled into alignment. During the planning visit, small marks were tattooed into my skin to indicate the exact position I had to be in on the machine's bench for the beams to hit the same spot every time. Precision was critical, and the radiographers were professionally focused on their target. I didn't doubt their ability to get me into position and to run the programme. But other things about the radiotherapy – such as my experience of it – seemed less skilfully thought-through. I became irritated and fixated on the spotted green smock they gave me ('That's yours to keep until the end of the treatment'). It was two separate pieces of cotton held together at the shoulders and sides by velcro. 'You can put this on in the cubicle in the waiting area,' they told me. I did. Then as soon as I was lying down on the machine's bench, one of the radiographers ripped the velcro patches on the shoulders apart and pulled the front down to reveal my naked upper torso. The smock kept me modestly covered for approximately twenty seconds between entering the radiotherapy room and lying down on the bench. It was to ensure decorum, I supposed. A leaflet about the treatment ended with an assurance that maintaining my dignity was important to the team. Even if it helps patients with breast cancer who aren't inclined to reveal their body, by the time they are on the bench, being naked is necessary. Perhaps it is more for the team's protection, so that they don't have to see the patient walk topless from the doorway to the machine. My modesty; their embarrassment? There was nothing about the situation that suggested the slightest likelihood of impropriety.

Either way, the green smock was a gesture rather than a solution. My dignity was left at the door of the treatment room each day, not because my breasts were revealed, but because as soon as I entered I became a loose component, a part the machine lacked, that had to be slotted into place to enable it to perform its function.

One of the two or three radiographers usually said hello when I walked in, but not always. They were already busy setting the machine up. I climbed on to the hard, narrow bench and lay down in the right sort of position, my legs elevated by a couple of cushions to prevent too much pressure on my coccyx, my arms above my head and my hands gripping a bar to keep me from moving them. Then, having pulled the smock down to my waist, two radiographers stood, one on either side of me, and called out numbers to each other over my naked torso, as they pushed and pressed a bit of me here, another bit there, not moving me, but nudging my inexact boundaries into co-ordinated perfection. The room was quite cool and usually their hands felt icy against my skin. No one thought to warm them before touching me. Once I jumped they were so cold. The radiographer said: 'Don't move.' 'Your hands are cold,' I said. 'Yes, but keep still.' Then, having fitted me into place and completed the puzzle set by the machine and my flesh, they called out to tell me as they went that they were leaving the room.

I was alone and had been made ready for the Elekta Linear Accelerator to perform its *danse macabre* around me. (For a week or so, before I Googled it, I naturally imagined it was an Electra Linear Accelerator, and wondered how the machine and its purpose made someone think of the grief-stricken, vengeful daughter of Agamemnon. It seemed no more apt than the baby seals.) Two massive arms were pulled out from the huge silver wheel set into the wall behind me, a third was already positioned above me. This one was circular with a mirrored surface in which I could see myself and the green line it projected on to me running vertically a couple of inches to the left of centre, marked by the indelible tattoo. It winked a green light as a small lens or portal opened and closed. The other arms were different. One ended in a large plain rectangle the size of a small coffee table, marked with black 90-degree angles at the corners of an otherwise invisible square. Apart from that it was quite blank, hovering over me, a slab, and like the rest of the machine, made of the same dull putty-grey plastic that computers used to be made of before they burst into colour (perhaps there will be a generation that remembers the putty-grey computer age being superseded by colour, as mine does the 1950s turning to the 1960s, or the door opening from a black-and-white Kansas to the brilliant colours of Oz). The third arm ended in a kind of thick crescent shape, like a massive herb chopper, or perhaps Poe's pendulum, though it was fixed to the movement of its arm and couldn't swing. The three cumbersome arms remained stationary over me, at my side and under me, then rotated clockwise or sometimes anticlockwise, until they came to rest with a different arm directly above me, while I lay perfectly still on the bench.

At the start of each treatment while the radiographers were setting me and it up, leaving me to my own thoughts, I wondered how to describe the machine. I never found a solution. Even looking at pictures of it online I've failed to make sense of its fangledness. It was a clumsy thing of parts, working in unison, but never summing up to make a whole. It wasn't designed to look like what it did, or for its use to be understood with just one look. It lived precisely where bland intersects with banality. The designer on the Terminator movies would have wept to see it. There was no external clue to whatever each part did, though I guessed the mirrored arm beamed the rays at me. If that was so, what did the other, blank arms do? The three arms moved around me, stopping and starting, humming sometimes, remaining still and silent at others, emitting a variety of clicks and whirrs, and suddenly reversing their circular movement around my body and under the bench as if the machine had taken a wrong turn. No one told me what was happening, and before the technicians went into their safety room it didn't seem possible to interrupt their measuring minds to ask what, exactly, it was doing as the arms moved or didn't. One small victory was asking them, as they left the room, to turn the bright ceiling lights off that were hard on my eyes. They did, but I had to ask them every time to do it. I gathered some part of Elekta scanned my insides, while others moved into position to shoot beams into my lung and lymph nodes, moving upwards towards my neck.

Then it did what was hard to determine. Sometimes it peeped for three or four minutes, and I supposed it was a warning that it was accelerating rays into me, but not always with a particular part in a particular position. I couldn't decipher any pattern or repetition in its movements. It stopped sometimes, as if pausing for a rest, for five minutes or more: was that when it was beaming me? Twice it stopped for longer than that, though I had no way of telling the time, and I was eventually told over the intercom that something had gone wrong with the computer and they'd have to start the whole rigmarole from scratch. I rather hoped the computer kept the glitch in-house rather than aiming the wrong beams at the wrong place in me, but I had to make do with the flat tone of their voices to allay that anxiety, as you look for signs of fear in flight attendants when the plane begins to wobble. Usually, it took twenty to twenty-five minutes to complete its staccato dance. The indescribable machine was overwhelming in its grey, looming blankness, its movement purposeful but meaningless to me, substantial enough to evoke a feeling of claustrophobia even though it didn't contain me like the tube of a CT or fMRI scanner. I had irrational moments when I feared one of the arms would collapse and fall on me, or that the bench I was lying on would suddenly rise up and crush me between itself and the mirrored arm. It was quite cold in the room and by the end of each session my arms were numb from having kept motionless for so long. I made another small improvement by wearing long arm-warmers, but that didn't improve the cramp. The first time I wore them, the radiographers laughed: was I the only one who felt the cold? But the one time I got on the bench forgetting the arm-warmers, one of the technicians reminded me to put them on. It was the nearest we got to a human encounter. Apart from the two more friendly radiographers, hardly anyone spoke to me except to ask my date of birth and address each session, to ensure I was the right person for the treatment. I suspect that rote Q&A tended to diminish my personhood in this machine-driven department. The daily repetition added to the sense that I was there, correctly numbered, a part that needed to be slotted in for the machine to be complete.

After a few sessions I stopped putting my pointless smock on and just took off my top and left it on the chair about four feet from the bench. The ceremonial ripping away of the front while I was lying down with my arms over my head was more disturbing to me than crossing the room naked from the waist up. It recalled when I went to Esalen in Big Sur and spent much of the time lounging in the natural spa baths built into the rocks looking out on the Pacific Ocean, comfortably stark naked in the sun. The radiographers wore neat fitted white tops with short sleeves over their trousers, and seemed a great distance from the 1970s frolic. If the youthful technicians were embarrassed by a few seconds of my mobile, aged nakedness, but content with my twenty-minute static nakedness on the table, I decided they would have to deal with it. They may well have thought that the brief covering-up provided the patient with that assured dignity, but it was just another formality, like my date of birth and address, that made me invisible. I put the lack of human connection in the radiotherapy department down to the fact that the technicians were dealing with intricate measurements that had to be done exactly right for each person arriving one after another for short periods over a long day. I'm sure it was tiring and tedious. But I didn't take to being no more than a date, an address and a package of flesh to be manoeuvred into the proper co-ordinates. I'd never felt like that during the chemo sessions, where the oncology nurses seemed to know that they were dealing with an individual, even if they were infusing a dozen people a day. If I sound grumpy and cross, that's how I felt going to and leaving the twenty daily treatments.

Perhaps, though, it was my mood that affected them. In order to get to the radiotherapy department I had to walk along the corridor that ran beside and was open to the general oncology waiting room. Everyone I know who has encountered that waiting room shakes their head at the memory of it. It's a huge space that disappears round the corner, with row after row of chairs, almost always filled, for a hundred or more to have their blood taken, while others waited to see their doctors. It seemed as I passed day after day that everyone was in a kind of trance. All these people with cancer, and friends of the people with cancer, waiting for treatment or to find out test results, resigned and passive on the rows of chairs. It was sometimes so full that people had to stand. Occasionally someone whispered to the person next to them, but mostly everyone kept a respectful silence. There was always a queue for the reception desk at the centre where the waiting room turned the corner. Behind and to one side of most of the chairs, out of the sitters' sight, was a large aquarium brightly lit by a bulb inside the lid. It was filled with a plastic shipwreck, and green plastic plants waved in the water thanks to a motor oxygenating it. It wasn't until the third day, the third pass, as I walked towards the radiotherapy department, that I looked hard, and established for certain that there was nothing alive in the aquarium. No fish, no seahorses, not even a water snail. It was a water and plastic under-seascape. Which was all right because no one looked at it. The bright, fishless aquarium that no one looked at seemed to fit in with the surroundings. There was no escaping the ready-made analogies. The ship of fools on an empty sea. The polite waiting for waiting's sake. Waiting for their turn in the anteroom of the afterlife with all eyes directed towards the electric sign that showed whose number was up.

The fully equipped, decorated aquarium without any fish probably had contained fish but they had died. Perhaps they'd given it two or three shots replacing the dead fish with live ones, but they all died. So now the tank was kept brightly lit and perky with no chance of dead fish floating troublingly on the surface, there just for the light and colour, which, even though it was in no one's eyeline, certainly made that corner of the waiting room brighter, and contrasted with the quiet forbearance of those who sat uncomplaining, whatever time of day I passed them. It became a matter to ponder while lying on the Elekta bench. Perhaps the aquarium had never had any fish in it. Had it been donated and it was decided the tank was quite nice as it was? Or had the accountants given the oncology department an ultimatum: lit-up seascape or fish? One or the other. No funds for both. Had the nurses put it to a vote while everyone sat and waited? Fish or seascape? I imagined one patient standing up and making a passionate plea for fish. He got a cheer. But the head nurse reminded them that a fish without a lit-up seascape would not make much of a splash. And, she added, if the powers that be say that the oxygen pump was only there to get the decorative vote, the result would be dead fish, which would be discouraging for children, or those with memories of fish they'd loved in childhood. The vote went overwhelmingly to the bright but fishless option. The patient who had made his passionate plea for a fish returned his eyes to the black-and-white number machine on the wall, which ticked each number to tell a patient their waiting was over. He looked down at the screwed-up paper in his hand and up at the number on the wall and realised that he'd missed his call. He got up to take another number. That fantasy took me as comfortably as it was possible to be through a death-ray session.

Once or twice, to see a doctor and to have blood taken, the Poet and I took our seats, and became one with the silent mass of cancer patients and their friends or family. I often tried to go past without looking, but it was impossible. I tried chatting to the Poet as we walked along that section but even looking away, there it was, the vast oncology waiting room which confirmed my growing suspicion that practically everyone has or had or will have cancer and will end up here waiting for the number on the machine on the wall to match the one screwed up into a ball between fingers and thumb. The much smaller radiotherapy waiting room was light relief. Some people nodded greetings and chatted. After all, everyone who was there came every day. You began to recognise faces and played the new guessing game: which one has the cancer? It wasn't always easy to tell. What was clear was the distinction between those of us who were having 'curative' radiotherapy and those who weren't long for the world and were having it to help with pain management. Some of the latter arrived in beds pushed by porters, patients, all of them grey of face and still, never looking about them at their surroundings. Others, more mobile, came having been delivered by volunteer drivers and sat grimly with various wounds and scars from surgery, breathing heavily, none of them looking around at the other patients waiting. We – the less ill ones – stole glances at these patients, those on their last legs or whose legs no longer held them up. Even the most buoyant and cheery patient in the radiotherapy waiting room must have seen the mirror the bedridden held up for us.

It's very difficult to get away from the oppositional thinking of good and bad, in cancer as in everything else. It isn't only the warrior metaphors: 'She's struggling with cancer'; 'She lost her battle with cancer.' All the explanations of my treatment, what it attempts to achieve and how it goes about it, describe the battle to erase the bad cells and promote the growth of good cells. Chemotherapy and radical radiotherapy (which means, I think, the maximum dose of cell-destroying beams my body can take) target the bad tumour in my lung and the affected lymph nodes (three are overactive, so far, north of the tumour). But neither the infusion of poison nor the killer rays, crude, unthinking hitmen, can tell the difference between bad cancer cells and virtuous healthy cells. So good and bad are killed off and damaged by both treatments. During recuperation periods in chemo, and for three months after the end of radiotherapy, where I am now, the good cells are given a chance to regrow, while the bad cells, it is hoped, can't (no, I don't know why, I may have been told once, but it didn't stick). The result is extreme fatigue because the body uses all the energy it has to rebuild itself. In radiotherapy the beams are as fine-tuned to their targets as possible, but for all the combined expertise and techniques of the physicists, clinicians and radiographers, they are also certain to damage healthy cells next to the tumour or the lymph nodes. Fatigue (I'm currently sleeping fifteen hours a day, and more) knocks me flat so that the body can use all its resources to work on regenerating healthy cells. The bad fairy's spell recuperated by the good fairy's amendment. Think Sleeping Beauty, dozing for one hundred years while briars and thorns grow dense around the castle, ensuring that only the best of the wandering suitors (princes, all) can cut their way through and plant a wake-up kiss on the slumbering princess. In the original case all the palace slept, too. What could a waking princess do when she discovered that all those devoted to her care, feeding, dressing, washing, teaching, had died long since? Enchanted princesses aren't equipped to fend for themselves when they wake, not even with a handsome prince in tow; they need the infrastructure of the palace and its denizens to make their waking life possible. When modern princesses wake up it's to a deliberately crippled NHS and princes who are as likely as not to have discussed the cost/benefit ratio of all that cutting back and concluded that making it through the briars just wouldn't be efficient.

My oesophagus, right next to a targeted lymph node, became inflamed in the last week of radiotherapy, and the ragged pain made it impossible to eat or swallow anything, especially anything with edges, for weeks. Although the pain has gone now, it's still difficult to swallow; everything feels as if it's stuck in my gullet, and my taste buds are playing a cruel game. Anything sweet tastes much sweeter and a lot of things, especially meat, are inedibly bitter. At Christmas the Poet and I had a lovely solitary day with work, DVDs of 1950s black-and-white B-movies, and a pheasant for lunch. But lunch turned out to be a matter of eating the insides of roast potatoes and leaving the elegant pheasant that tasted only of bitter aloes on the side of my plate. I was the cat that got the brandy butter but not the Christmas pudding.

A few days after treatment had finished, the area on my back where the beams that entered through the front of my body made their exit started to show signs of radiation burn. The skin went deep red with flaky patches and was dotted with painful nasty scabs. I resisted a Job-like soliloquy requesting that the Lord explain what I'd done to deserve this and settled instead for moping and muttering: 'What the fuck else is going to happen?' I spoke to the Onc Doc on the phone, rather than the Lord Almighty (consultants are the Lord's representatives on earth, anyway), who told me that these days burns were very rare and that I must have a particularly sensitive metabolism. Hydrocortisone cream would soothe it and, he hoped, prevent it from getting infected. I basked in the light of my remarkable metabolism for a bare nano-second before realising the message was basically: 'Tough luck. Get over it.' Not all that different from the Lord's reply to Job. 'Then the Lord answered Job out of the whirlwind, and said: Who is this that darkeneth counsel by words without knowledge? Gird up now thy loins like a man; for I will demand of thee, and answer thou me. Where wast thou when I laid the foundations of the earth? Declare, if thou hast understanding.' The hydrocortisone ointment has stopped any infection and calmed it, but it still hurts and itches, one and the other, hard to say which at any point, though the area of damage has grown smaller and paler. Another permanent side-effect is the worsening of the mild scarring of my lungs, which was already there, but now makes getting up the steep stairs of a Cambridge terraced house like a pilgrimage to Santiago. These side-effects, including the fatigue, which seems to be getting worse (as well as others I've been lucky enough not to be so sensitive to, and have avoided), can continue for weeks after the end of treatment, and, as a Macmillan brochure – one for every cancer anxiety that arises and my first stop before Googling – tells it, can stick around for months or even years. Short of dying from them (people do), the unwanted toxic results of treatment are considered worthwhile badnesses, a trade-off for the greater good of destroying the rapidly reproducing cancer cells and upping the chance of living X or Y months longer. A month after treatment ended, I am more tired for longer than I was (if I allowed my eyes to close, I'd be fast asleep over my MacBook Air in a trice), and I curse anyone knocking on the door for causing me to go down and then back up the stairs. Still, my burned back is healing. I have no idea what all this has to do with clubbing seals, but they keep popping their heads up, blinking dolorous eyes at me.

So treatment is over and there is nothing much to do in my cancer-world except wait. Sometime in February or March, I'll have a scan and see what all the poison juice and darts have effected. It's like peeping over the edge of the world while remembering you've left your spectacles on the kitchen table. Or more accurately, like eating custard and ice cream while watching endless hours of *Inspector Morse* in the hope that your chemo-brain will have wiped at least one episode from your memory bank.

After waiting that long week for the results of my post-chemo scan, the answer to the hovering question about the effect it had on the tumour in my lung and the affected lymph nodes was much the same as most eagerly awaited answers to important questions. Inconclusive. As I'm learning to expect, nothing very decisive has resulted from the treatment. The tumour has shrunk a little, but, Onc Doc said swiftly, it was small to start with. The lymph nodes too have decreased a little in size. There was neither excitement nor disappointment in his manner. It may be that he has the same air of studied neutrality in his everyday life, when eating a delicious meal or going over the top on a rollercoaster. Or, more likely, it is for work purposes alone, in order to prevent overexcitement or crashing disappointment in patients with unrealistically high hopes or fears. I imagine that his 'but the tumour was small to start with' was intended to prevent disappointment at the seeming slightness of its reduction: a small reduction in a small tumour is not to be sneezed at. It seems I am to think that the cancer that can be seen hasn't got worse, indeed it has improved, and if I were the right sort of character, I could take heart from that. To me, being the sort of character I am, it means I've got cancer ('So what took you so long to arrive?'), and I won't not have cancer, but as the Doc said at our first appointment, a certain amount of time can be added to my life by the treatment (two to three years instead of perhaps fourteen months) before the symptoms begin and the dying process starts. I smiled and said, 'That's good' in a way that I hoped showed I hadn't got any unrealistic hopes up, and that I was grateful for his, the nurses' and the radiographers' efforts. The team. And, of course, I am grateful. I try to feel grateful.

As far as I understand it, the main problem is with the spreading of the cancer via my lymph nodes – this is what happens most commonly with lung cancer – to brain, to bone, who knows where? When I asked, the Onc Doc said that they hadn't seen any new cancer sites, but they couldn't know if there were cancers too small yet for the scan to pick up. 'We can only see what we can see with the instruments we've got.' I assume that the cancer spreading minutely through my body, like microscopic pig-iron in diminutive goods trains, is the reason, even with treatment, that my life expectancy is still only a fairly abbreviated two to three years. It's a travelling cancer sending its cells here and there, so that only when they have taken root and grown can they be seen, by which time, I imagine, new invisible seeds will have been planted elsewhere. Etcetera. Still, if Onc Doc's super cool is not just professional and he maintains his chill when hurtling down Kingda Ka, the world's highest rollercoaster, then I might be wrong and I should rejoice at least somewhat in the diminishment of the visible cancer cells. Anyway (I'm working hard on attitude here), it must be better than the tumour staying as it was or getting worse. So, as planned, the radio-therapy has begun. First the measurements and then the daily dose. Each treatment, twenty minutes of zapping. A month of treatments, Monday to Friday with week-ends off, throughout November. (Here comes Melville: 'Whenever it is a damp, drizzly November in my soul; whenever I find myself involuntarily pausing before coffin warehouses . . . ')

There is a sense of things going to plan, but no magic. There's nothing to be done except wait while the medics keep everything as contained as possible with radiation, and see whether, three months after the end of radiotherapy, the tumour has reduced, and, more important, if the cancer has spread and grown visible. There was no new mention of that original two-to-three-year prognosis if I had treatment. I didn't ask, because I was fairly sure from his manner and what he didn't say, that the prognosis hadn't improved, even if it hadn't got worse. In other words, I will continue to live with uncertainty and my inability to do anything about it, the condition I've been trying to wriggle away from all my life.

It's absurd to complain about the uncertainty of life expectancy – we're all just a breath away from the end of our lives – but it's especially absurd from someone in their late sixties. For almost a year before the diagnosis, I'd been plagued by thoughts of the possible not-so-far-in-the-future depletions of body and mind of one of us, me or the Poet. The future played out, in my mind, with each of us having innumerable strokes, serial heart attacks or one of the other less decisive but nonetheless disabling illnesses of old age. Turn and turnabout I'd have in my mind one of us debilitated or dead, then the other. The urgent question was: which would I prefer, to be the carer or the sufferer? The dead or the survivor? How long before one or other of us could no longer live in our two-storeyed house with its steep stairs? When might it be necessary for one of us to be looked after by professionals in a care home? We've lived together more or less for sixteen years. Sixteen years ago, the future still seemed a long time ahead, even if to our young selves back in our thirties, either of us in our fifties and now sixties would have seemed as old as we could imagine without picturing mobility aids and incontinence pads. Getting myself to imagine us as our young selves might imagine us was enough of a jolt to make the mind accept the present not-at-all-terrible reality of time and the body.

But within a moment of accepting the reality, I returned to its consequences, which is to say the deteriorated future of our ageing bodies and minds. The fact was that the depredations of old age were no longer so far ahead that they could be dismissed as 'sometime in the future'. The fear, as my late fifties turned into my early sixties, grew to become a fear of certainty, rather than uncertainty. I wouldn't say I preferred the certainty, but I knew at least where I was. Then to have the diagnosis of cancer dropped into my model of the future, to be told that with an effort I *might* live for another *two or three years* brought back the uncertainty, so that both conditions, fact and speculation, each at their most unpleasant, now existed side by side, as equals.

Can I learn to live with certain uncertainty, or uncertain certainty? I know that so many other people live with exactly that, from illness or poverty or war, but that thought doesn't help. I'm no better at tolerating unresolvable uncertainty than I was when I was fifteen and going to live with a perfect stranger while receiving letters from my former chums, inmates of the Lady Chichester Hospital, cheering my good fortune and wondering how I was getting on in my new life.

I can't remember a time when I didn't provoke myself with impossible thoughts. To begin with I wouldn't have known which were impossible and which not. But, curled up in a favourite dark place (I've always longed to be behind those deep-red velvet curtains where Jane Eyre sits on the window seat, leafing through Bewick's *History of British Birds*), or lying awake playing mind games in bed, you find out quite quickly that the imagination comes to an end in a deeply unsatisfactory answer to the question being put. Even so, I continued to try and tease out meaning for the words and the facts about life I discovered as I grew older and read more. The daily and nightly probing began around the age of six or seven, always ending at a wall or a miasmic fog in my brain. Looking back, I'm sure that it was tied up with my readings of *Alice's Adventures in Wonderland* but especially *Through the Looking-Glass* – which easily brought dizzying thoughts to mind. What if the rabbit hole never ended? How to deal with the White Queen's 'Jam tomorrow' which never comes today? And of course, the practice of believing six impossible things before breakfast. Which, if it did nothing else, at least told me that impossible things were there to be thought about.

Most things became easier the more I did them, but my mental investigation of the creeping idea of infinity never got any further. Yet I couldn't stop poking my metaphorical tongue at the metaphorical loose tooth, rocking it back and forth until the pain went beyond interesting and pleasurable. I'd devote every ounce of my being to the task of understanding the endlessness of infinity, as if one great push (birthing spasms, the fanciful Disney lemmings' forward rush over the cliff to oblivion) would crack the problem open and I would find perfect understanding in the pieces that lay at my feet. I worried that the endlessness of infinity must come to a stop somewhere, because it hurt my brain to try to imagine that it didn't. Later, more grown-up in years though not in the things that worried me, I learned that the universe wasn't infinite. Somehow. Then where was the edge of the universe? But that meant another universe, another edge, more and more, and there I was, back to infinity and dizzying brain ache. I simply couldn't fathom, and for some reason thought I needed to, the parameters of the unending. I was using the wrong language, it turned out. Maths was invented to grapple with concepts that metaphor made murky. But I couldn't think in that vital language. Just wasn't my thing. So clinging on to the figurative to save my life, I vaguely grasped that the end of the infinite might be where death started. That required more probing. At first, when some knowledge of death's ubiquity came to me, the main concern was the catastrophe of my parents' death, hotly followed by adventurous orphan fantasies (Tick-tock, Cap'n Hook, here comes an awfully big adventure with gnashing teeth), and a narrative which developed but never ended because I fell asleep.

Both infinity and death were beyond me. They defeated me, and although I came to know that everyone was subject to death, it was some time before the penny dropped that I, too, would eventually be part of the seething crowd of everyone who dies ('I had not thought death had undone so many'). Melodramatic accidents were story material, but an ordinary death at the end of my life was an absurd proposition, and so remote as to be hardly worth getting a sweat up for. Even so, I'd lie awake trying to imagine being dead just as I tried to imagine stepping off the end of infinity.

It was easy enough imagining myself being dead, settled peacefully in my coffin, everyone sobbing into handkerchiefs, no unseemly snot in evidence, for their poor beloved dead child, but soon enough I realised that I'd got in my own way. Death is the end of you. Of me. There is no being dead. The body, the coffin, the tears were for those who were still alive. Without a notion of a holiday-camp heaven, something I seem never to have had, I was left with a new and special kind of endlessness, like infinity, but without you. By which I meant me. You and then not you. Me and then not . . . impossible sentence to finish. The prospect of extinction comes at last with an admission of the horror of being unable to imagine or be part of it, because it is beyond the you that has the capacity to think about it. I learned the meaning of being lost for words; I came up against the horizon of language.

So it's not as if I haven't thought about death, yours, theirs, my death, all the time, now and back then. Like Gabriel in Joyce's 'The Dead', I've imagined 'the vast hosts of the dead'. And in my childish way, I understood

Gabriel's vertigo: 'His soul swooned slowly as he heard the snow falling faintly through the universe and faintly falling, like the descent of their last end, upon all the living and the dead.' But until my cancer diagnosis and the cautiously calculated prognosis last summer, death in all the forms it had come to me, or as I had worried it, was a description of the unreal. There has been grief in my life, though very little compared to many. A great grief, the loss of one of my oldest friends, my first husband and my daughter's father, only came on me in 2011. A loss to me, whether we saw much of each other or not, of his being in the world. Your inevitable imagined death isn't properly a grief until you look at it from the point of view of those who will remain alive without your being in the world. When the Poet expresses his sadness and forthcoming grief, it hits me as if I were him and suffering his loss of me. It is both a lesson in empathy and an indulgence in narcissism. I will, by then, not be suffering anything. Will not be. The pain and sadness that engulfs me at his distress is projection, a mirroring of another soul. Perhaps it is an exercise in the reality of love. How else can I conceive of my own death even though I now know it will happen sooner rather than later? I did make one request to the Poet from beyond the grave: 'I don't much care about the funeral arrangements, but if I'm going to be buried, I want to be tucked up in a winter-tog-rated duvet. It doesn't have to be exquisite winter-snow-goose down, though that would be nice. But I need a duvet. You know how much I hate being cold, and especially cold and damp.' The Poet put his foot down. He hates waste and whimsical dishonesty. 'You won't be there to feel the cold and damp,' he said. Tears came, just up to but not spilling over the lower lid. Mine. His. Sometimes it's hard to tell.

'I *know* I won't. But now I want the promise of a duvet.'
'Double or single?'

Nevertheless, the excruciating terror of the fact that I am in the early stages of dying comes regularly and settles on my solar plexus directly beneath my ribcage (called my coeliac ganglia, from which the sympathetic nerves in charge of the fight or flight response radiate, or called anxiety, or, if you prefer, my third chakra). There the terror squats, rat or raptor, its razor-sharp claws digging into that interior organ where all dreaded things come to scrape and gnaw and live in me. Still, so far, unabsorbed. Undigested. Dropping in on me, like the weighted lead of grief, when not expected. Give me medication, however unnatural, at least to round off the knife-edged talons scraping away at me. Give me some distance, some respite from this kind of pain as you do from the pain of cancer treatment, or cancer itself, or a broken wrist. It's not a lesson I need to learn. I've known and recognised the underlying psychological causes, some of them anyway, enough of them. I own up to them and I really don't need this solar grip to remind me of my fear. Death feels your collar when you're going about your business almost as if nothing has happened, and when you are idling, wondering what there is to think about. Whoa, hang on, missus, the world has come to an end.

Negativity is my inclination, whether biochemical and/or environmentally produced. Looking at death as negativity, of everything gone, an absence, I get the image, from *Psycho*, of Hitchcock's (or Saul Bass's) shot of swirling bloody water draining into the plughole and transmuting into a teardrop in the corner of Janet Leigh's open, dead eye. Her face crushed against the floor tiles, she can neither gaze into the abyss nor have the abyss stare back, because even the abyss is non-existent in the non-existence that used to be you. The abyss is merely a penultimate state of the ultimate.

I have 'non-small cell lung adenocarcinoma'. I'm mystified by the term. By the negative term for its opposite. Non-small. A robust sort of cancer, then? Why not 'large' or 'quite big'? It reminds me of Poe writing in 'The Pit and the Pendulum' that his protagonist 'unclosed my eyes'. Was 'opened' on the very tip of Poe's tongue, but he couldn't quite make the reach? I sense a pantomime audience howling 'Opened! For god's sake, Ed. Opened!' Or did Poe choose this peculiar usage to unsettle the reader by throwing a net of the uncanny over the horrible moment of vision? But that can't be the reason for the medical term 'non-small'. Is it simply large-celled, but courtesy/custom/delicacy requires the euphemism? What need? *Undead* has quite another meaning. Where does this linguistic black hole get us? Non-alive, non-pretty, non-excellent. And up pops *non-existent*, just when I don't need it. Hey nonny-no. In my third novel, *Like Mother*, the main character was called Nony for short – a baby girl born without a brain (although the narrator of the book). Non-existent. Nonny no.

One of the things I was very clear about immediately after my diagnosis as a canceree was not wanting to be dropped into the 'victim' arena. Not worst of all, that awful designation, which chases us whatever we are doing or misdoing, being 'on a journey'. When I began this memoir I anticipated with dread, and hoped to bypass, the crushing moment when I would first be described as 'being on a journey'. Might have been King Cnut, for all the good that did. Quite a few people ignored me, as is their right, and jumped in anyway, launching my boat, giving me a pat on the back to get me going, firing the starter gun, swimming alongside me for a while, hoping I would stay the course, wishing me strength for the road I travelled, all of them knowing but not actually saying that journeys do end, that's the point of them, and we all knew where this journey ended. Right at the start I was in a funk about the avalanche of clichés that hung over my head in a bucket that we would all, me included, tip up to cover me as if with pig's blood at my first and last prom. (How do you do? The name's Cnut, Carrie Cnut.) Clichés exist because they once worked brilliantly. They helped to universalise the intractably private, to keep a distance between what people wanted to say and couldn't. They must have been alive then. Now they are either the deadening end of meaning or party favours to be played with. For some writers they are a springboard, perfectly placed to be rejuvenated, to renew or cut through their general use as thought-concealers. If people reach so readily for a cliché, it's because there's something they can't say, or even think. When Beckett or Nabokov twists a commonplace into an oh-so-considered sentence, it too does the work of the uncanny. The too well known as unknown. I fucking love clichés.

Still, there is also the matter of just being accurate, taking the straightest route to the meaning you want. I am not on a journey, I repeat, testily. But as each of my treatments ended I found it grew harder to escape the platitude. The good cell/bad cell dichotomy of the body hosting cancer is difficult enough to avoid. The phoney spiritual analogy has become inevitable, everything that happens for more than a split second is a 'journey'. It's not our fault that time works for us in the way it does, or that the linear accelerates our lives. We 'journey' as we read books, watch films, look back at our past, imagine the future, even mindfully try to live in the always and only present moment while thoughts of what was, and is still to come, crowd our minds. Otherwise there's silence, and that's an option. Though not much of one for our narrating species. Can we even get dressed without a before and after, a beginning and end? Starting with your socks instead of your knickers doesn't alter the fact of the matter: undone to done. And then the reverse. One, two, buckle my shoe. It's inescapable. From one state to another, how can the journey not come to mind? That's the price of living in time. Why should I mind so much? Why should I mind so much now? Because journeys end?

What's strange is that the multitude of journeys we are all deemed to be on have become coupled with optimism, no matter that for most of human history a journey was always begun with the knowledge that it might not end well or in the right place. Ships were wrecked, brigands stopped and stripped pilgrims in their tracks, disease ended any thought of destination or arrival. The first time I experienced a journey with no destination was when the bailiffs came and took our stuff away, promising to return to evict my mother and me from the flat in Paramount Court. My mother, rising to the occasion, took my hand and dragged me along the streets, shouting at me that now we were destitute, and were going to live 'under the arches' in Charing Cross with all the other tramps and beggars. I knew some of the tramps who had a regular route between the Rowton House workhouses and I hailed them as they arrived in Tottenham Court Road, where

I played. But we weren't heading directly to Charing Cross to claim our space: we were wandering. It was raining. I remember the dark pavement, watching my feet walking (my head down), the splashing of the falling rain, and for the first time being out and walking but without a destination. Before that if we went out we were always going somewhere, if only to a shop and then to return home. This was quite new and terrifying, we were just walking. Homeless, with nowhere to go. Of course, eventually, after my mother's rage and fear had been walked off, we returned to our flat, still in possession until someone came and sorted my mother out with social security and a bedsitting-room in Mornington Crescent. Walking in the rain still makes me feel bereft, even though it's only an echo of a fear that didn't happen.

But these days, being 'on a journey' assumes that you will reach your destination to a hero's welcome, a happy ending, an apotheosis, something having been learned or earned, and approved. The slightest of efforts by an individual or a group is crowned with the completion of an inner journey that the actual journey (often not a journey) has nothing to do with. People wear T-shirts printed with their favourite charity's slogan: 'Let's kill cancer', 'Bring a homeless dog happiness and love.' They run in circles, or cycle to the ends of the earth, Swim the Channel, the Atlantic Ocean, several lengths of the local pool, climb Mount Everest, a Munro, a plastic wall, spell more words correctly than anyone else, and in November write a novel or grow a moustache. The money you 'earn' will provide goods for the needy, a drip in the stream of scientific research funds, and the effort you make will buff up your character. A journey seems always to be for the better. It ends in insight or excellence or positive change. But can Rolf Harris, formerly beloved entertainer, now convicted sex offender, be said to be on a journey as he slides down the fame snake to a cell in Stafford Jail? Still, if he makes a statement on his release, it's likely he will tell us that he has been on a journey and learned lessons, perhaps even got himself straight with God, in readiness for the final journey. Has anyone willingly grasped the hellish consequences of their actions since Don Giovanni's fevered acceptance of his murdered victim's invitation to dine with him in hell?

> Who lacerates my soul? Who torments my body?
> What torment, oh me, what agony! What a Hell!
> What a terror!

Much as I hate it, the journey – that deeply unsatisfactory, often deceitful metaphor – keeps popping into my head. Like my thoughts about infinity, my thoughts about my cancer are always champing at the bit, dragging me towards a starting line. From ignorance of my condition to diagnosis; the initiation into chemotherapy and then the radiotherapy; from the slap of being told that it's incurable to a sort of acceptance of the upcoming end. From not knowing, to 'knowing', to 'really' knowing; from being alive and making the human assumption that I will be around 'in the future', to coming to terms with a more imminent death. And then death itself. And there is no and. Maybe it's just too difficult to find a way to avoid giving the experience a beginning and an end. Except that it's never over, cancer, until the fat lady pops her clogs. No one is ever cured of cancer, except technically. Even if I were to pass the magic five-year survival post, or go into remission, the possibility of a return of the cancer cells will always be there. Binary oppositions turn spatial. Whichever way I refuse to call it a journey, the pattern of a voyage is etched into every event. How can I avoid the idea that I am at the least on a journey from Big C to Big D (as everyone is, although the letter of the first stage may be different)? Why do I want so much to avoid the notion of a pilgrim progressing? What if I try it the other way? I'm standing still while the tests, diagnosis and treatments pass by me as if on a belt. This is not outlandish, the supermarket checkout, or *The Generation Game*, where the prizes roll along in front of you on a conveyor belt and you get to keep those you remember – a teas-maid! From first inklings, it is all outside me, moving at its own pace, while I observe attentively. Or like the journey I made by Amtrak around the US, watching the swiftly or sluggishly passing scenery through the window as I sat dreamily on a train. No, trains have destinations. Perhaps I'd better think of myself as sitting idly at a station, hanging out, while diagnosis, treatment and so on arrive, stop and depart. Me, I'm not going anywhere. Just watching the passing show. But it's such an effort, wriggling away from the platitude while the journey taps her feet in the wings knowing where she belongs.

The end of the journey doesn't come until you either die cancer-free of something else, or die of the effects of a regeneration of the cancer cells. Good and bad; from here to eternity, and from eternity to here. But I have been *not here* before, remember that. By which I mean that I have been here; I have already been at the destination towards which I'm now heading. I have already been absent, non-existent. Beckett and Nabokov know:

> I too shall cease and be as when I was not yet, only all
> over instead of in store.
>
> *From an Abandoned Work*

> The cradle rocks above an abyss, and common sense
> tells us that our existence is but a brief crack of light
> between two eternities of darkness.
>
> *Speak, Memory*

This thought, this fact, is a genuine comfort, the only one that works, to calm me down when the panic comes. It brings me real solace in the terror of the infinite desert. It doesn't resolve the question (though, as an atheist I don't really have one), but it offers me familiarity with 'The undiscovered country from whose bourn/No traveller returns'. I've been there. I've done that. And it soothes. When I find myself trembling at the prospect of extinction, I can steady myself by thinking of the abyss that I have already experienced. Sometimes I can almost take a kindly, unhurried interest in my own extinction. The not-being that I have already been. I whisper it to myself, like a mantra, or a lullaby.

In between the metaphysics, the memoiring and a previously unknown addiction to vanilla ice cream, there's been some doctoring, testing, diagnosing and everyday hovering and waiting. Plus standing by for the new grandchild, whom I don't suppose I'll know for very long, scoops of the vanilla ice cream and statistics that will no more keep me alive than the eggs, cream and vanilla pods. Still, I'm not looking for a reprieve, except that I'd like to get to know yet-to-be-born Flora/Edie/Jessie/Rosie or whoever she will eventually be who seems to have been doing upside-down headspins. More fun probably than being thumped through the narrow corridor towards the intolerable light in the birthing pool, where, as I write this, she's hanging on by tooth and claw to stay in the previously cosy warm pool she's been in these past nine months.

About four months after finishing the radiotherapy, it turned out it had not finished with me, and I found my mild breathlessness becoming much more urgent. Quite suddenly I couldn't climb a flight of stairs without stopping to catch my breath, I couldn't walk from my bedroom to the adjoining bathroom two steps down without finding myself in a coughing fit; and then I had my first panic attack. The more I coughed the more I gasped for air, the more I gasped for air, the faster and more shallow my breathing became. I could feel the 'floor' of my lungs rise higher until there was no more room for any air to be taken in. Without doubt, I was dying of suffocation. It wasn't a metaphor, it was an inability to breathe, to take in air; and I knew that I wouldn't survive this attack.

I did survive, of course. It took some minutes, though probably not as many minutes as it felt like. Gradually, the coughing died down, and the floor of my lungs dropped so that I could take in more air, until I realised I was still breathing and not about to die. I waited for ten minutes or so to allow my shocked body to calm down. This happened three times when I was on my own, and once when my daughter was here. I described it to the Poet, but I knew that he would understand it as a 'panic attack', a great but not life-threatening discomfort. An episode of distress, where dying and suffocation were just dramatic words that I co-opted to convey the horribleness of my experience. What I learned from speaking to Grace, who came from the local hospice to see me, was that the radiotherapy had inflamed my lungs, already scarred from the original pulmonary fibrosis. That was a known risk, but as it was later explained to me, the degree of the scarring and inflammation was much greater than had been expected.

A couple of days later I fell down the two steps into the bathroom and ended up in A&E at five in the morning with a broken wrist. Even I could see the comedy: two terminal illnesses and now a broken wrist. *And* I had my travelling bottle of morphine to save the duty doctor the trouble of writing up a prescription. The following day, Grace gave me information, comfort and a plan of action at least for the panic attacks. A swig of morphine (a measure that was between a sip and a slug) before I started to move, a hand-held battery-operated fan to blow air into my face (this has no medical basis but has been found to lessen the feeling of suffocation in many people, and it did in me) and a couple of reminders to tell myself: to let my shoulders drop and raise my head, and to remember that this had happened before and I hadn't died. The panic attack had so frightened me that I would have recited *The Very Hungry Caterpillar* backwards if it had been shown to help fend them off. A later fall left me with three broken ribs as well.

The Poet and I, love each other though we do, needed some respite; he from worrying about my falling and breaking something every time he goes out, me from feeling a hopeless, helpless invalid, incapable of doing anything for myself. I was given a week at the wonderful palliative care home nearby, better known as a hospice – a word that causes a shimmer of death to run up and down the spine. I got lots of work done in spite of people popping in to introduce themselves and offer resources and massage, and the Poet got a rest from free-floating angst for a few days. The hospice people help with everything, co-ordinating the activities of the suited doctors and specialists who seem to have very little idea of what anyone else is doing. Within days of my key-worker palliative nurse being on the scene, all sorts of things were arranged and achieved. Railings for the stairs, classes in breathing technique, medication reviews that discovered the dose of nortriptyline I was taking for depression was too high and could be causing the postural hypotension that makes me lurch all over the place and lose my footing so that, in spite of the railings, I'd managed the broken wrist and the three broken ribs. So now (start counting) I've got pulmonary fibrosis, lung cancer, postural hypotension, pain with any kind of movement – like breathing – from the three broken ribs, and difficulty typing or lifting anything heavier than a small pillow. Next stage down, the steroids I'm taking to prevent inflammation have turned my face 'cushionoid' (new bit of technical learning here), which means rounder and fatter at the bottom, a shape my usually long face has never known, and my limbs weak. I'm like one of those young secondary characters in a Victorian novel who aren't long for this world and have to spend the day resting on a chaise-longue taking deep breaths from time to time.

Though I'm not young, I am not all that long for this world, it seems, but it's hard to pinpoint how or when.

The full lifetime's worth of radiotherapy I was blasted with inflamed the fibrosis far more than was expected, but the chemotherapy, a horrible experience in itself, seems to have stopped the development of the tumour. Now I'm more likely to die from fibrosis than cancer, which might have gone into remission, but as deaths go, they're much of a muchness (or as my overemotional GP said, 'They're both such terrible ways to die'). As it stands, I will be fighting for breath with both of them, although the wonderful palliative care nurse calmed my fears by explaining the steps they take to calm my body, so that I fall into a sleep and then a coma and die unconscious and in some comfort with the aid of intravenous doses, regularly increased, of fentanyl and morphine, drugs I take now in other forms for pain in my neck, the bust ribs and the broken wrist. Dying of lung cancer can be treated the same way, so the terror of death has been soothed to the fear of blank nothingness into eternity. A nonsensical fear as soon as you stop to think about it. Though think about it I certainly do.

What no one can help me with is time. *When* am I going to die? How long have I got? I don't feel what you'd call well now, but everything that hurts or is uncomfortable is the result of a side-effect of some drug or process intended to slow down the progress of the tumour or fibrosis. As soon as you ask 'How long?', you can see Onc Doc's eyes shifting into eidetic motion to remember the figures for death in either case. He offers me statistics, smoothed to take in the doubleness of my disorders. He can say between one and three years, assuming I don't get an infection that my white cell system isn't strong enough to prevent from turning into fatal pneumonia rather than a common cold. The uncertainty is real. Onc Doc's skills are essentially statistical. Reading papers that include and conclude from other studies the mean average life-time chances. But I'm not a statistic. As an individual, who knows? A friend of mine in his eighties had received chemotherapy and was feeling much better; along with his doctor, he was expecting a few more years of life, but he died two days ago from a heart attack, brought on in part by the stress and damage of the chemotherapy, itself a life-threatening procedure. I no more know when I'm going to die than you do. Statistically, it's now better than it was: between one and three years. It doesn't feel so urgent. The Onc Doc has partially signed me off to the fibrosis doc (although the organ is the same, fibrosis and cancer are two entirely different expertises, requiring two separate specialists), and then another range of statistics will come into play. But in reality, who knows? The oldest person I knew, my former father-in-law, died last week, aged 99, after telling several people he would like to die, that his arthritis was too much for him; he went to sleep and stopped breathing. That seems, though what do I know, as gentle and civil a death as I can imagine.

In the meantime, logic and time aside, there's the two-year-old grandson waiting at home with a friend, while his mummy has now had his baby sister. He had been knocking on his mum's belly and shouting, 'Come out, sister, we're waiting' (possibly another reason for her hesitation). But I don't feel so gloomy about being dead long before his long-term memory has kicked in. I'll be in some books and photographs and a few stories he's been told. And some hazy memory, story mixed with reality. That's what really distresses me. Idiotic to feel weepy about someone who has already given so much pleasure not having 'real' memories of you. Who does have real memories of their early youth? Still, the tears well. There's narcissism for you.

There's nothing stoical about any of this. I've thought and felt it through in every possible way, and I can only make sense of the sadness because it is sad. Sad for me. Sad for others too, but in a much vaguer, normal, only-to-be-expected sort of way. Certainly I wouldn't, like my former father-in-law, want to attend the funeral of my child. If I'm being over-logical about it all, repressing the pain, I can't see it. I feel the sadness even more sharply, now that the new girl child has been born, at the idea of missing knowing what they will both be like, later, what they will become. But I can't stop myself remembering that this is how it is supposed to happen. How many grandparents live to see the full development of their grandchildren? So the news medically is relatively good, but somehow, I'm still managing to mope.

———

If it were a race, the first man home – except for Iain Banks who won the trophy by a mile – would be Oliver Sacks (announced 19 February – died 30 August), with Henning Mankell (announced 17 January – died 5 October) a close second. Lisa Jardine won a race of her own, staying shtum publicly, her death a surprise except to the few who knew. So Clive James (announced May 2011 – ?) and Diski (announced 11 September 2014 – ?) still battle it out for third place. In the other kind of race, last man standing, James and Diski would be meandering towards first and second place, Sacks and Mankell having already taken third and last place. These are the writers who within the last year or so (nearly five years in James's case) have publicly announced their forthcoming death from cancer, of one sort or another.

It's a delicate balance, this publicising of one's cancer. The public's interest is fixated on when each of them will die. For some reason cancer is the disease of choice for public tongue-wagging. It has that something, that *je ne sais quoi*, not just death, but how long known beforehand: how will she die, should she choose to try for a longer life by accepting treatment, or settle for palliative care which at its best is a comfortable death without pain. What Francis Bacon called 'a fair and easy passage', which I used as the title of a TV play written and broadcast long ago. An announcement of forthcoming but more or less certain death by a public figure opens our eyes to death, the one that is coming to us all. I don't know why but cancer is the definitive illness. People run in circles and slide down towers to show their solidarity and 'earn' money for research. But there is an edge. James wisely jokes about it, but 'they' don't really seem to want a cure or long-term relief for cancer sufferers (unless it's a family member or a close friend): it seems to spoil the purity of the tragic. No one so far as I know has written a column or agreed to an interview to announce that they have flu, or arthritis in their left knee, and how the medication is going. It's not that flu or arthritis couldn't be made interesting – it all depends on the writer – but in the cancer cases, it isn't the quality of the writing that's being judged, but the murky details of the illness that will remove each candidate from the board, and if it doesn't the audience will feel cheated.

'I bet you've found faith now,' believers wrote to Christopher Hitchens when he announced he had terminal cancer. He insisted he hadn't. I'd never been envious of those who believe in an afterlife until now. It would be so much cosier than dissolution. She's gone to the next room. Nope, can't manage it. She's gone to dust and rubble. Gone nowhere. No *where* to go to. No *she* to go to it. Much easier to be convinced you will be met in Elysian Fields by a thousand virgins, or drink from fountains of Manhattans. I can't even get close to what they call faith, though I quite see Pascal had a point; and so did Wittgenstein (though quite wrong globally) when he said: 'Go on, believe! It does no harm.' I don't and won't, and there it is.

Doubtless there are writers or public figures who have recently been diagnosed with cancer and have chosen not to mention it. Quite likely, among those of us who've written the 'I've got cancer and I'm going to die, watch this space' piece are some who are grateful for a subject that will indeed last them a lifetime – provided the lifetime is relatively short. But already Clive James has had to apologise for not yet being dead and explain that doctors have produced a medication that can keep his kind of leukaemia under control. He seems to feel that his readers are wondering if the whole thing was maybe a hoax to get him more attention. He did say in August 2015 that he was living on borrowed time, though he could understand the impatient foot-tapping of his readers. It's obviously lost him the 'who dies first' race, but in the 'last man standing' race he has all to play for. 'Which writer lived the longest and wrote the most columns and/or books after announcing their forthcoming death?' I offer this as a question to *University Challenge* or a 'What comes fourth?' puzzle on *Only Connect*. Jesting as hard as he could, James said: 'I am waiting for the next technological advance which I hope will enable me to live for ever.'

I am also alive, having announced my lung cancer (with a side attraction of pulmonary fibrosis: two fatal diseases – I don't do things by halves) in September

2014 in the *London Review of Books*. And I too have been knocking back pills that Nice has licensed only for specialist use. Or I was. It took four weeks to build up to the full dose, which was three pills three times a day with meals. The aim, as with Clive James's medication, is to keep things on an even keel. No cure is expected, just a slowing down of the deadly events going on inside me. My cancer is sitting where it was, but the fibrosis has been having a private party since the course of radiotherapy livened it up no end. (My fibrosis doc was consulted by my Onc Doc as to whether I should have steroids to prevent the deleterious effect of radiotherapy on fibrosis. He said he had no worries about that.) So, as of my last scan my cancer hasn't gone away but is keeping quiet in its corner of my left lung, while the fibrosis situation is an unknown until I have a scan at the end of November, but is much worse than when I first wrote about it. How many lung cancers equal a rapidly inflamed fibrosis of the lung? I stopped taking the pills after a month or so because they made me sick, nauseous and sleepy. The Papworth doctor said that was OK: there was another pill I could try, but after that 'There will be nothing else we can do for you.' My pills might keep me alive for a year, the consultant said, with a doubtful side-to-side movement of his head.

Unfortunately, this three-meals-a-day thing is not a habit I've acquired in my time. There is a wall of misunderstanding between the Poet and me.

'I can't eat lunch, I'm not hungry.'

'You don't have to be hungry, just eat enough lunch to take the three pills with.'

I'm stupefied at the thought that it's possible to eat when you aren't hungry (though there are apparently people who can), just as the Poet is stupefied at the notion that you have to be hungry in order to eat. I snack and, if the Poet didn't cook, wouldn't eat what anyone would call a 'meal' for days on end. The first time the 'You must'/'I can't' debate happened the winner was, of course, me. I agreed to a small bowl of rice with sweet-corn and peas. Who couldn't manage that? I managed about a dessertspoonful, taking the pills as directed. Within twenty minutes I was vomiting the whole mess into the kitchen sink – couldn't make it upstairs, not enough breath. There is nothing I dislike more than being sick, though I've recently discovered that a panic attack that involves being unable to take in any air runs a very close second. I have no more to say about it. Except that I did show the Poet I wasn't just being faint-hearted. 'Exactly,' he said, 'it's psychological. You were sick because you wanted to show me that you couldn't eat if you weren't hungry.' This debate – is throwing up a physical or a psychological response to three pills and a small amount of food? – went on for a while without resolution. Though if the Poet had the slightest inkling of the extent of my dislike of vomiting – you could call it a phobia – he would never have suggested it was voluntary in any way. My stomach had to be well-lined with food, so that the extremely potent pills could be digested and not rejected by my body, designed as it is to keep poison *out* of my system. So now, waiting for the next and last pill, we're in a bit of a quandary.

Do I want to live another year or so, or do I want to throw up, feel ill and eat when I haven't the slight-est appetite? That is a new alternative. I have to digest it before I can begin to answer it. A decline caused by fibrosis or lung cancer is very unpleasant. But throwing up that night, and the prospect of stronger and nastier medication, left me thinking about the balance. Worth another few months? Worth it for whom? How miserable will these extra months of life be? What the docs call quality of life measured in qualia. Versus, I suppose, no life at all. I had believed that Francis Bacon's 'fair and easy passage' was a real possibility. But I no longer trust the hospice key-worker's assurance that the dying process can be made painless. There was an unpleasant incident recently when I was told I could have a week's respite (for me and the Poet) at the local hospice, and ended up leaving ten minutes after I arrived – they had no record of my request (granted twice: the week before and the day before) for a single room. A bed was available in a four-bed room, but a need for privacy and the degree of my depression made that impossible. I wanted a private place to cry where no one would be upset or ask me to stop. I was polite, I hope, but very disappointed. Later in the evening a doctor from the hospice called and told me that they 'don't provide respite care' and couldn't possibly guarantee that there would be a room for me when the time came for dying and palliative care. I had thought that both things were precisely the point of the hospice movement. I was shaken and distressed. The doctor later phoned my GP (not me) to say that she thought she might have upset me by being too definite in what she'd said. Well, we all have our bad days. But who the bad days affect matters too.

People offer me things to live for. (Another TV quiz show?) 'But what about the grandchildren? They're worth living for, aren't they? And family and friends?' But finding what is good about life makes their loss all the more miserable, even if you know there will be no you to miss anything. In this long meantime, dying sooner rather than later can be upsetting. Additionally, how much do I want to be dependent on others for my everyday life or, indeed, for finding a reason to stay alive a little while longer? Missing a few months of feeling awful, being dead, versus not missing those months of feeling awful. Dead, at least theoretically, is the less painful of the two options, assuming that dead equals not being at all. Whatever terror there is lies in the present fear of dying, not so much of death. The stoics tell me that I've been 'dead' before, prior to my birth, and that was no hardship, was it? Back to Beckett, I think. So that's how I am at the moment of writing this. But of course it's more complicated than that, more complicated than is allowed by the linear business of writing one word, one sentence, one paragraph after another with the intention of being coherent.

I have a feeling that if I describe my daily life, 'the reader' will react with sympathy for the blank, sedentary existence my condition causes. The thing of it is, though, that my daily life is (with obvious exceptions) very close to my idea of a perfect existence. The day usually begins with the Poet and me having tea in bed. I also have porridge or Weetabix (or did before I revolted over taking the awful pill). Every third day my fentanyl pain patch has to be changed. Not cancer pain but long years of chronic pain in my neck. Then we generally moan about the news, our dreams, the awfulness of now compared to then, the awfulness of then compared to now. An hour or so of this and the Poet gets up, washes, spruces himself with one of the strange, expensive perfumes he has on his bathroom shelf. Not that he's a narcissist; well, he is a narcissist, but he's also, I think, chasing the scent that is his spirit smell. He has about a dozen that are close, but none of them so far is quite *it*. His *totemic* smell. So further investigations and purchases are intermittently required. Knize Ten and Géranium by Dominique Ropion for Frédéric Malle rate very highly, but there's probably a scent out there somewhere that is more essentially *him*. This is much the same attitude as I have to clothes. I look now at a handful of catalogues or I look online, but when I got around, in shops, just sometimes there was a garment that had been patiently hanging on its hanger waiting for me to find it. It's a mystical thing and also expensive.

When he's finished with the shower, the shaving, the unguents, he gets dressed. So far so uninteresting. At this point, he writes on a whiteboard on the back of the door the events and times of the present day. For the last few months, I have lost all sense of where we are in the week. Every day for me now is usually Monday, or sometimes Sunday, occasionally Friday. You know that certainty one has about time and its larger chunks? Well, I don't have it any more. Since the treatment started, I have to check (and often recheck) the day at least and sometimes the month. Still, not a really big deal, though unsteadying when I thought I had that cracked around the age of six or seven. While the Poet eats his breakfast in the kitchen – no porridge for him, but homemade granola, lightly home-stewed berries and plain yoghurt (shop bought, I'm glad to say) – I begin my day, which involves straightening the bed and getting my laptop on my lap. The Poet goes off to college or the library and my day's work starts here, between an hour and three hours usually, either on these memoirs or the monthly article I write for a Swedish paper (in English, to be translated into Swedish. Strange). Work finishes when it finishes, with me tired out, physically exhausted, or I discover that I have closed the lid of the laptop and, without thinking, declared that's that. The Macmillan book of cancer treatment says it can be as long as two years before the exhaustion goes, and that doesn't take account of my original pulmonary fibrosis. And then the big decision of the day: do I put away the laptop and sleep, or do I have a shower and get up? It makes no difference except that it feels silly to shower, clean my teeth and dress, and then take everything except a T-shirt off and get back into bed to sleep for between one and three hours. As differences go, it's vanishingly small. Either way I end up back in bed, exhausted. More if I've washed and dressed, and much more so than before my cancer treatment started. Of course, there's the wash and dress first option, then get undressed and get into bed to work (but actually having to sleep off the tiredness of having got up in the first place). So many options, so few options. And so many ways of operating them.

Eventually, after teaching, or poking around in the University Library, or writing references (when do the poems get written?), the Poet returns, for lunch or supper which again I have to eat, against my better judgement, in order to take my pills. Then I shower, or wash, if I haven't already, and dive in slo-mo into a djellaba thing or baggy pants (not baggy enough since the steroid weight-gain catastrophe). I read, we watch some TV and chat, and then, around ten, I go to bed, having taken my handful of antidepressant pills, which serve me better as sleeping pills. End of my eventfully uneventful day.

Tomorrow is, or so the Poet insists when it comes, another day, but I usually say 'Sunday' or 'Friday' in answer to his question or my own testing. My two-year-old grandson, when asked a question he can't or doesn't want to answer, says after a moment: 'Ella'. Which, I think, serves for the 'Fuck off' that I've been forbidden by his mother to say in front of him. I might adopt this ploy, and each instalment of this memoir/cancer diary will be filled with the word 'Ella', from top to bottom of each page. That's a pleasing notion. Restful. Dear keyboard please repeat copied word – 'Ella' – to end of memoir. Cf.:

> Have written more than a hundred pages and not got anywhere yet. My calendar is getting confused . . .
> Don't think I can go on. Heart, head – everything. Lolita, Lolita, Lolita, Lolita, Lolita, Lolita, Lolita, Lolita, Lolita. Repeat till the page is full, printer.

My calendar is frighteningly full, to me. It no longer involves the arrival of couriers delivering my pills or the district nurses taking blood to see if the pills are damaging my liver; the senior psychiatric nurse who has brought a fold-up wheelchair in case I'm taken with the idea of a wheel round the Fitzwilliam or the Botanic Garden. The geriatric psychiatric consultant comes every two or three weeks. On her last visit, she decided there wasn't much point in changing the pills around, adding this or upping that, because my depression is 'well-founded'. This distinction is new to me. It presumably replaces the now disgraced endogenous/exogenous types, abolished by the latest *Diagnostic and Statistical Manual of Mental Disorders* because, I suppose, they found a couple of descriptors they like better. 'Well-founded' and . . . actually, I don't know what the new word is for 'endogenous': 'She's just like that,' perhaps, or 'idiopathic', which is also the description of my kind of fibrosis, which might have been caused by working in asbestos-lined factories or spending quality time with certain birds, but wasn't. It means 'don't know how that got there'. Another use for 'Ella'. Why have you got pulmonary fibrosis? Ella. Do you want to be wheeled round the Fitzwilliam? Ella. Meaning I'd like to look at a couple of pictures I especially like, but don't want to be wheelchaired. Maybe I'll Google the recent divisions of depression later on, between naps. 'Well-founded' has a double response from me. On the one hand it tells me that I've a perfectly good reason to be depressed (dying sooner rather than later from two incurable diseases and haunted by the memory of my former GP saying, in a torment of pity and tactlessness: 'Oh Jenny, they're both such terrible ways to die'). I presume, if I weren't depressed by that, I would be diagnosed as being in pathological denial or psychotic over-optimism, but no one has ever suggested that I suffer from either of those. Sometimes other members of the Cambridge health team turn up: occupational therapists who have organised grab rails for nasty spots where I might fall and break something more than my wrist; outreach workers from the local hospital or hospice who have also given me a course of six foot massages. Very nice, but I don't know what I've done to deserve them. I even have my very own friend. Sourced from the Poet's many pals (who I like but usually don't go out with him to visit or 'dine'), my new press-ganged friend pops around once a week or so and we gossip. That's very nice. I enjoy it. Then there's my daughter Chloe and her frighteningly large family – two small children and partner. Vast by my miniaturist standards. One child good. More than one, tempting fate. But also very nice. I get more breathless but less bothered by it. I get out of the house just once a week when the Poet drives me to the top of our road, to have my hair washed by my splendid young hairdressers. They are sweet and kind and seem to have substituted 'ah bless' with 'definitely'. 'My hair is a real mess.' 'Definitely.'

So having given up on the vomit-making pill, there is one other: 'There's nothing else we can do for you.' Doc language for 'You've failed us and you'll just have to die, which is not our speciality, so goodbye.' Or as my grandson would put it, 'Ella'. My breathing has got worse and I can't get to the car without waving an electric hand-held fan in my face and swigging on liquid morphine. A pain in my left side has suddenly ratcheted up times ten. I'm a bit of a wreck. Actually, a super-sized wreck. I presume that the three stone I put on within two weeks of starting steroids make me all the more breathless and less able to pick myself up when I fall. I'd never thought about it before but the weight you are is the weight you carry. Literally. I suppose all this is what most people experience. It's either dying suddenly in a car accident, or having a helicopter fall on you, or one of your many organs that manage your many other organs going out of kilter and spinning the whole system into a whirlwind heading deathward. I'm perfectly sure that there are quiet deaths that creep up on you gently at a decently old age, or thanks to skil-ful palliative care, and that I must hope for that sort of ending.

PART THREE

Spray It Silver

> I am not writing volume three of my autobiography
> because of possible hurt to vulnerable people. Which
> does not mean I have novelised autobiography.
> There are no parallels here to actual people, except
> for one, a very minor character.
>
> *The Sweetest Dream*

I can't get away from that paragraph. It feels like a well, bottomless; time to hold your breath before you hear the distant splash of a coin somewhere down there. It's the careful donation of kindness. The passage is a kind of labyrinth: not to hurt 'vulnerable' people. They must be real, they must be alive, or why bother with it? So we know that what follows is a sort of non-fiction. That wouldn't surprise us: Doris often used people and situations in her writing without feeling the need to alert readers. Even those not particularly vulnerable might still have cause to feel upset, since no one is named yet anyone could be implicated. Doris is protecting some people but giving them due warning, and warning others who are real and might take it that they are included. Could there be a more simple way to warn certain people, and cause many blameless others distress than these three sentences?

What judgements are being made about whom? Here is a sticky business. She is protecting some (real-world) people by not writing about them. But by saying that she is not writing autobiography she is telling us that something happened. (What kind of something? What is she telling us about? Sex, politics, her version of some truth that has been confabulated?) Only when they are dead are the letters here allowed to be read. That is the meaning, the weight of having the last word. Something happened, or someone did something – and those of us who are innocent will have to remain in ignorance, never knowing who did what. The accusation doesn't go away. Nor can the magnitude of the 'truth' contained here now be known, or checked and then questioned.

I can't help comparing the author's note in *The Sweetest Dream* to the letter I found on the table that morning, for me, furiously accusing me of emotional blackmail for wondering whether she liked me, or even wanted me in her house. But what is to be done? If fear or abandonment are arresting your heart, can you forever live without an answer, pretending it doesn't matter? Or in a multiple blindness, can both parties know the question and the need but never speak of them? Apparently you can. That is what's so odd about the author's note. It only has one meaning for a particular person. But its tentacles of worry reach out to include everyone. When a child is told to stand in class and accused of something they haven't done, a fountain of guilt springs instantly from the vastly overstocked pressure cooker – god, the relief and terror – and whether or not you are guilty (and sometimes I was), the spume rises up from the passive wicked place inside you. There's always more, of course, the dark deep place being fathomless, but this release is some lightening of the load both for the genuinely guilty and for the free-floating anxiety that longs to be locked within the innumerable tentacles. Who did it?

Another Sufi story comes to mind that Doris used often. A bowl of rice has been stolen and the possible culprits are made to stand in a line. 'We shall see who took the rice.' There is a silence and then the Mullah speaks and points to the villain. 'It was you.' But Master, how did you know? 'Only you touched your beard for fear that some rice might have stuck to it.' Not a really convincing story. All the components must be in place already: rice, thief, beards, knowledgeable Mullah. Good thieves would not touch their beards. It's a poker story: watch out for the tell. But those loaded with free-floating guilt will touch their beards too. Injustice is written in to the story. Someone stole the rice, someone was hungry, they all had beards. A wisdom story must do better than that. Doris's author's note declares: I will tell the world who the guilty ones are, but not until they are safely dead and cannot answer back. And then there is that single 'very minor' character. Why? Why does such minorness get his or her reality mentioned? Are we to scour the pages? Is it worse to be a minor character than to be an important one protected both by sound and silence?

I feel as if there ought to be a machine perhaps made of paper clips, or rubber bands, that this piece of prose could be put through and it would come out the other end making simple, complete sense. We are supposed to have one (I call it a brain although some care to call it mind) but it is always going wrong. When I read those lines, the less sense they make, and the more my word-untangling machine seems to tangle words and everything in sight, Yes, that, and that, and even this. So I give it another go. Read it fast, read it shallow, read it deep, don't read it at all but keep it under the pillow on my bed; doesn't matter. Shut the book and think of something else, hope for a sweet dream, but anything would do.

More and more I hear Alice moaning along with her dream and her mirror companions, Humpty Dumpty, the Red Queen, the vanishing cat: all that terrible caterwauling from most of them extracting every last drop of juice from the words readers have forced them to speak.

They speak the puzzles a new language presents to them. They are easily distracted by etymologies, rhymes and the lack of precision of the language that Alice was once so sure of. Alice, of course, is somewhere else, in Wonderland or Looking-Glass world, and both she and the others explain just what she means by the words she has used all her life, words which have consistently been responded to as if there was no problem about them. If that author's note were an Alice character, she would have the same problems as the others do with language and the White Queen does with hair pins. Here comes Alice's entourage again – and again – to tell us that some things make nonsense, or at any rate only make sense to the teller and the story. And that, I'm afraid, we just have to put up with.

The author's note in *The Sweetest Dream* is more than a metafictional trick, like John Ray, Jr, PhD's foreword to Nabokov's *Lolita*, the outsider's perspective on the mad and repellent Humbert Humbert telling us it's all right to sit back and enjoy the perversions of others. But this is Doris Lessing: not playful, not one for fun, the writer, knowing how her book is going to be received, instructing her readers how to read what has been written by her in the following pages about the atmosphere and events of the middle years of the twentieth century, although there is the further warning: 'Some events described as taking place at the end of the Seventies and early Eighties in fact happened later, by a decade.' So the book is fictional – it's *The Sweetest Dream* – although at least one of its characters might, if they read it, recognise themselves: it's not too hard, even given a hair-colour change or the fact they wear high heels rather than trainers. But it's non-fiction, too, in her use of timings. It's OK, apparently, to make events that occurred in the month of May 1962 happen, after all, in 1982. She doesn't explain very clearly. The 1980s have their own problems, their own pleasures; but for Doris, not wanting to hurt feelings or wanting events to make more sense for her 'novel' means reorganising time. Decades have their own time and feel.

In one way she is setting up the reading of the book as a *roman-à-clef*, or throwing a cloak of visibility over those fictional characters, who we should suppose ghost-like, unnamed, not creatures of flesh and blood. It is not the third volume of her autobiography although I can't remember anyone ever suggesting it was. But it isn't a history book either because placing events a decade earlier or later makes the 'events' she speaks of things which like bubbles drift along and burst here or there, having no particular moment or effect in their reality, or in 'Doris's' reality, depending on where your shoe falls. Nothing is affected when they burst. The more I read it, the more this author's note perplexes me with its triviality, like the trail of sweets to the witch who wants to cook and eat the children for supper: witches get hungry too, but are devious in their method.

Novels, you can do pretty much what you like with them. That's what they're for. Who's going to tell Melville what he has to do in *Moby-Dick*? But authors' notes I take very seriously. I imagine, for example, those vulnerable people she speaks of, now more or less my age, those of us who undoubtedly did sit around Doris's table in the mid-1960s, reading the author's note and then the book itself. 'Phew, it's not about me, then.' 'No, that dress was as black as a starless night and she's ruined it by making it an idiotic green.' Or: 'Is that what she really thought of me, back then?' Or: 'I'm glad I'm not one of those vulnerable people who isn't in the book.' Or: 'Fuck! That very minor character is me. Me, a very minor character.' *Ceci n'est pas une pipe*. It's not even clear if we can rely on the author of the author's note being the author of the book. Someone has to take responsibility for this written object I hold in my hand. And with that, Alice and I set about looking for a garden with a tea shop nearby: we've been assured a tea party is going on somewhere, and lie down to have a nap.

And Doris herself, who I take to be the author who has written the book and the note, what to make of her? There's a bouquet of nuances in those two brief paragraphs. There are some quite threatening tones, written by someone who knows the power of words – words she can choose either to she speak or keep to herself – because of the way they can hurt, distress or disturb others. Watch out, keep your place, or I'll have the world – or at least a lot of people's lives – thrown into the flames. But there's generosity too, because – knowing the hurt she could cause – she has forsworn writing the dreaded third autobiography. And then again, that generosity comes with a reminder and perhaps a warning to some of the 'vulnerable' that she has such power over them. After all, the simplest way not to hurt people is not to spread words she might if she wanted to write but won't be. Or perhaps all this is a form of apology to the vast majority of her readers who must be disappointed if they really were waiting for Volume 3 of her autobiography. She is explaining why. Or she is explaining herself to those who, knowing her those fifty years or so of hearing the gossip around the table, enjoyed the tales and stories as much as anyone. Those who could point out which of her friends the characters were, though they have been developed for the purposes of the story. Nothing was straightforward about Doris, as writer or gossip. It doesn't make her very different from other writers who take what they need from people and events that suit their needs for their fiction.

I can remember several vulnerable people in the 1960s, some of whom sat around Doris's table, friends of Peter and friends of mine. Others were continents away. Some of them I still know. Some of them are still vulnerable. Some of them were Peter and me. Doris knew that writers, some more than others, never keep things to themselves: they take a morsel of her, make his eye colour different, turn a her into a him.

No, what I really want to write about is a short walk I regularly made from a bus stop in Shoot-Up Hill in Brent, across the road and along a street called Kingscroft Road, to a house, the top flat of which Doris had bought when the Charrington Street house was compulsorily purchased by the local council, and after the flat she had moved to in Maida Vale turned out not to be to her liking. According to Google Maps it is about a three-minute walk, which surprises me. I thought it was longer. I don't remember what date she moved there, but during that time I was running the free school for intractably difficult children, studying at a teacher training college, and then working full time as a teacher in Hackney. I lived in a small flat of my own in Camden under some joint ownership arrangement, which is now nothing more than an infuriating dream-scheme for young people trying to find somewhere cheap of their own in which to live. My three-minute walk happened over several years that took up most of the 1970s. I often made the trip at the end of the school day in Haggerston, or from my flat in Agar Grove, to see Doris, usually weekly, invited for tea or supper, or for lunch at weekends. Whichever place I started from, it seems that a bus (I always used buses rather than the Tube if I could) took roughly the same time. Between thirty-nine and forty-seven minutes with a clear road. Even in the mid-1970s a clear road was hard to find on Shoot-Up Hill, which ran the dull length from Kilburn to Cricklewood, and upwards to northern places I still haven't heard of, changing its name as it went along, perhaps just to keep bus passengers on their toes, in the hope that it might eventually transform into something along the lines of a garden paradise for those who stayed the course. It's really the Edgware Road, and the nearest thing to magic is the Three Wishes pub some way after Brondesbury, where I got off.

I've lived long enough and done enough things to be certain that the first year of teaching and the first months of baby care are the most tiring things a person living a non-extreme-sporting life can do. I was always bone-tired; there was no baby until 1977, but the free school and my probation year at Haggerston had me hankering for my bed at home in Agar Grove rather than tea in Kilburn. But I don't think that explains what I'm wanting to say. I'm just chipping it in there for those who prefer practical explanations. From a long but not unrestful journey on the bus, I'd press the buzzer or bell or whatever it was to stop the bus, and step down from the platform on to Shoot-Up Hill's pavement. The very moment my foot made landfall, the anger began as if the pavement and the soles of my shoes had closed a vital circuit. Nothing fierce, just a familiar nudge, an awakening, a quickening, a sleepy stretch making ready.

A few yards along from the bus stop there was a zebra crossing. Maybe twenty or thirty steps. At each foot-fall the anger increased. Instead of swelling, it recoiled, contracted, showing its steely strength like a hooded cobra, coiled around itself while arching its head, pull-ing it back, sucking in all the energy it needed to make a lightning-fast strike. The slow build-up, followed by the equivalent of a hundred-yard dash, using stealth and speed to perfection to kill its prey, or protect itself from the accursed god in the garden of peace and quiet. A little like that, but not good enough. The foot on the pavement, the irritation as both feet felt solid ground. The moments before I jumped off the bus knowing it was going to happen, because it always happened, and things that always happen on cue can never be prevented by trying to stop them. And things you don't want to think about in order to keep them away always do what they do because the knowing is no more under your control than an infant waking up hungry and crying out for milk. Let's drop the cobra. Let's call it a thing with-out will or the need to protect itself or to feed itself, or with any animosity towards its creator because it is a nothing. Buddhists would call it a 'sensation' to make it no more or less significant than an itch on your nose while you are trying to meditate. Being too hot or too cold, feeling hunger, feeling dull, all just sensations. Notice them, name them if you will and let them go while you take the calm, quiet road back to the present moment. I've found that can work for quite difficult things like pain. I've got a broken wrist at the moment. If I call it a sensation, go towards it, breathe into it, frag-ment it, breathe it out and away, I can manage to type with nothing more than a different sensation in my right wrist from the one in my left. But the walk from the bus stop to the zebra crossing never failed to be what it was. Never impressed by my playing mind games with it.

Rage. A rage that stank like garbage in a wheelie bin on a sweltering summer day. But it started slowly, like the serpent in the garden condemned to move on its belly, to have its head crushed by the human and to strike the human's heel. By the time I was at the crossing it had curled itself into the tightest of springs. As a rule it lived nice and quiet down in the viscera, somewhere dark-red and moist that thanklessly produces or regulates some hormone or other to keep a body going in a nice homeostatic fashion. The heart beating like the grandfather clock in the kitchen, all the blood and guts, humble organs, keeping time. Controlled and controlling. This three-minute walk – probably a bit longer because I'm a slow walker and I would deliberately constrain my steps in the hope of getting the Spring Thing back under my control.

That walk, like any repeated event during which one's mental pathways are etched into the body by the brain, was always the same. I don't know when I first noticed it as a pairing of mind and body. The moment when you say to yourself, this always happens here. I always have this feeling at this point; it begins here and grows as I step towards Doris's flat, cross at the crossing, walk along Kingscroft Road, see the grubby pebbledash of the house, walk to the door. Another door. One side and the other. But with an opening device that lets you in, if the inhabitant of the flat wants to see you. Only one side of the door occupied. Not so interesting, but as I walked into the empty corridor a rage so dangerous that I sometimes thought I might have a heart attack from the anger that shot up from its coiled self in Shoot-Up Hill, as it sprang powerful and metallic but always kept inside. Not really dangerous, honestly, an anger that afflicted only me. Another door. This time the right sort. Me on the outside, Doris inside. I knock, although she knows I'm there because she buzzed me in. Doris getting up, probably interrupting a sleeping cat on her lap – Grey Cat dead by now, replaced by another whose name I can't remember. And the reader seeing both sides of the transparent door, two people, each hesitating and taking a deep breath, who really don't want to see each other, but were designated by some higher force to stay in contact, to be a family, Doris's obligation, one of her tribe.

Everybody leaves home, almost everybody. How you do it depends on the times and one's own experience. Although I'd lived with plenty of uncertainty by the time I was nineteen, leaving Doris's after four years was very frightening. I seem to be made more anxious by experience rather than more confident. I wanted, and for a while got, a place of safety. After a dismal, crazy, wrist-cutting time in the bedsitting-room I'd taken over from Olwyn Hughes, Ted's sister, I began to decline, in spite of my cunning plan to spray everything silver, as the linings were. (My first day there, as we swapped ownership, Henry Williamson told me, just as he was leaving after tea with Olwyn, the 'big secret' that T. E. Lawrence was killed because he was riding his bike dangerously fast after a call from London to take over the British Union of Fascists. 'You are a swallow among the starlings, my dear,' Williamson said to me – at least I wasn't an otter among the badgers.) For the next two years or so I was in a variety of psychiatric units, and for me these were all places of safety. Regularity, a schoolgirlish gang of ill-disposed young women, no responsibilities and twice-weekly sessions with methedrine and its friendly syringe, and the shrink telling me I was worthless. It gave me no future, but a safe place to wait and see. Despite the clean sheets, crazy nurses, friends, enemies, dramas, everything an institution can provide along with the expectation that I and the others would act out, the time eventually came when I saw that I couldn't really spend the rest of my life rattling from bin to bin. I overdosed again and was sent by R. D. Laing's colleague Aaron Esterson to an experimental group therapy clinic, where we spent all day in differently constituted groups working out our various problems with ourselves, using each other as exemplars. I lived during that time in a druggy flat in Covent Garden (on National Health benefit) and took all the chemicals I was offered, fortunately without dying, as some had. It was all a matter of luck, or some fierce inner determination to survive no matter how much I insisted I had no interest in being alive. I suspect the latter, though I'm loath to admit it. Even now I have a sense of shame at having survived to my late sixties. Everything I did looked like a lurch towards death, yet everything in my life continued. I overdosed with some seriously lethal barbiturates in a solitary room in Great Portland Street only to discover that the methedrine I'd previously been injecting myself with was in fact an antidote to barbiturate poisoning. I took the cure before I took the poison. I felt I shouldn't be alive, and in common with my headmaster, that I was always 'falling on my feet' though it was never my conscious intention.

So the acting out and the drugs passed me by and I got hooked up again with Doris, who, hearing I'd given up drugs, offered me the one-room flat in the basement of Charrington Street, while I worked as a secretary and made a pitch at becoming the 'normal' person Idries Shah said I had to be before I would be accepted as a student of 'the Work'. All very well, it seemed, but it was hard enough being an impossible teenager, how was I going to manage to act normal – something I'd had no experience with at all? Not since I'd been born. One thing all the comings and goings had achieved, however, was adaptability. I could put on a performance that seemed good enough to convince most people. The problem was that I had no idea what this 'normal' was that I was supposed to achieve. A secretary. Take shorthand, type it up, make cups of tea, look busy when there was nothing to do, be treated like a snail in the middle of a wet pathway. Doris seemed to think these were the kinds of thing Shah meant by becoming normal, and perhaps they were. 'Carry your bags, ma'am?' he asked as we were walking to a nuclear shelter (an unused underground sewer pipe) we were going to stay in as an experiment set up by the University of Swansea. When I said thank you but I could manage by myself he said: 'Do you think I'm a male chauvinist pig?' I was too embarrassed to answer this by-then ancient evasion. Others around me were shocked, and knowing from Doris how these conversations were supposed to work, I imagined that I was being given a chance to think through my attitude to sexual politics. I certainly don't think Doris would have approved of my allowing the conversation to end with: 'No, but I'm quite fit enough to carry it myself, thanks.'

This was Doris, a woman who had played whatever part was necessary to get her where (London) she wanted to be and what (writing) she wanted to do. In Salisbury,

Southern Rhodesia (now Zimbabwe) she had left two small children, a boy and a girl, with her divorced husband, and married a member of the Communist Party, an exiled German, with whom she had her youngest child, Peter. When she split up with Gottfried, she took Peter, aged two, and the manuscript of *The Grass Is Singing* on a plane and landed in London, staying with all sorts of hospitable post-war people with sometimes tragically spare rooms, who helped to look after Peter while she wrote and went to meetings. The last of these lodgings was with Joan Rodker, whose son Ernest, about ten years older than Peter, was at St Christopher's School. Joan was hugely energetic, running the party organisation practically single-handed and keeping Peter out of the way while Doris wrote and had affairs. 'The trouble with Joan,' Doris once explained to me, 'is that she never had very much luck with men.' Meaning that she, Doris, had. And surely, part of that analysis was that Joan was devoting herself to Peter, whom she was very fond of.

At seven or eight Peter went to St Christopher's too, though I don't understand how either Joan or Doris was earning enough money to pay the considerable fees. Joan worked at the BBC as a drama producer, and Doris was living on advances for her next books. I met Peter when I was eleven and had been sent to St Chris by Camden Council to get me away from my mother. He was known as Fuzzy. He'd just come back from a visit to Germany to see his father, who had had his hair cut in an erect German military crop. We never got on. We argued a lot. It was encouraged in class, but Peter had developed a pretend grown-up style which had come about from trying to keep up with all the political and literary types he was mixing with at home. They just ignored him or laughed generously, not taking him seriously. It made him as I recall pompous and self-important. When he was wrong Doris and her friends never corrected him or explained, so he would make wild pronouncements, and I was not kind or thoughtful enough to leave them alone at school, where he was with his peers not indulgent socialists.

Peter is the great enigma in the story of Doris. He actually *is* the story of Doris, both in her youth and in her old age. It's very hard to know how to present the two of them as the years went by, how to describe the dyad they made and which locked them together more and more grotesquely for the rest of both their lives.

―――――――

Peter Lessing died in his flat, of a heart attack, in the early hours of 13 October 2013, aged 66. His mother Doris Lessing, died four weeks later, on 17 November 2013, aged 94, in the adjoining house. An interconnecting door had been cut into the shared wall and was always left open. This very nearly tells the story of their lives as mother and son, in the sense that we know our planet is part of our universe, but there remain gaping holes of incomprehension that no one is going to be able to fill no matter how much detail their story is told in.

Peter was the child Doris took with her in 1949, along with her first finished manuscript, *The Grass Is Singing*. The two packages are always mentioned together. The manuscript was in the suitcase she carried, they say. The child is always noted, but in these mini-biographies or profiles, left to tag along. Did Peter hold Doris's hand, walking carefully, or follow behind her, or did he run on ahead, holding on to the rail, descending the metal steps from the airliner to the tarmac of his new country that everyone at home called 'home'? He was only two, how much sense could he have made of anything? By the time we are two we have been taken to many places: a visit to Auntie, shopping at the grocery store, a trip to England on a plane. Perhaps the tone of voice with which the adult announces the visit is the main clue to the import of what is happening. In my mind's eye, I have Peter tucked head first under Doris's free arm, as if he were swimming down to land, but kept safe in his mother's clutch. In the other hand she held the sort of small, shabby suitcase that pulp fiction illustrators give to people running away from their lives – to heroines with gumption, or plausibly handsome yet morally flawed young men. The suitcase holds the protagonists' future. The man uses his free hand to get ready to light a cigarette, pulling a silver cigarette case from his pocket. The woman obviously doesn't have a free hand. Her suitcase holds a few bits and pieces of clothing that are quite unsuitable for the new climate in which she will be living, but the manuscript of that first novel takes up most of the room. It will turn out to be the beginning of a career that ends not long after she wins the Nobel Prize for Literature. In the male version of the suitcase I'd guess at several shades of silk stocking samples, one of which will probably be used to strangle the life out of some lonely but restless woman, who at the moment hasn't the slightest idea of the man descending the steps to try his luck in post-war London. There might even be an inset, a small cameo of her in a neat shirtwaister, looking through the kitchen window, out on to a neat garden, thinking of something far away while she does the washing-up.

I mention these two puffs of fantasy to emphasise that I'm not attempting anything like a biography of Doris or Peter Lessing, still less my own autobiography: I'm writing a memoir, a form that in my mind plays hide-and-seek with the truth. It contains what I imagine and what I remember being told. Absolute veracity is not what I'm after. That man with the suitcase of stockings or murder weapons didn't exist, as far as I know, and won't be given another thought, although in a different format he might become a very Satan. Nor will I be chasing along Internet corridors and byways, or settling in for an afternoon in the British Library in order to verify the date and the details of the flight. I have no idea how people disembarked from a plane. It's very unlikely that Doris descended the steps into her new country (old 'home') in the way I have described. But there was an airplane, a woman of thirty, a small boy and a typed manuscript; and although in many cases when I write about Doris, I was present, I wouldn't dream of suggesting that I am offering a factual life of anyone, apart perhaps from myself – and there is nothing so unreliable or delicious as one's rackety memories of oneself. Some of my recollections may be tainted by time or others' slanted tellings or photographs, and my memories are no more and no less likely to be precisely accurate than yours or hers. I'm saying only that I was there, or was told first hand, and have remembered things thus and so, which might make what I recall a mite closer to the facts of the matter.

Doris Lessing left behind two ex-husbands, Frank Wisdom and Gottfried Lessing, and the two young children of her marriage to Frank. Men do this all the time – desert the family, shall we say, in one form or another – but we assume, partly because of sloppy, ill-considered thinking and partly with some element of truth, that the wrench is too great for any but the hardest-hearted woman. Even then, as with Ruth Ellis, there is an evil, compelling genius – David Blakeley, murdered by her as her only escape – or, as with Myra Hindley, an evil, compelling 'mad' genius, Ian Brady, virtually taking over her soul by making her do the most unimaginable harm to innocent children. Women's crimes or even misdemeanours go to the very spot where the meaning and value of 'woman' balances the murderous testosterone of masculinity and rescues the world from chaos.

When Doris's obituaries were being updated, in the days after she died, I was phoned by a journalist who wanted me to speak for the case that Doris had not deserted the children when the marriage broke up: that Frank Wisdom and his sister (another archetype: the malign half-sister or stepmother or surrogate mother) had embargoed Doris from seeing them, and that somewhere in an archive there is a letter from Doris saying something of the sort. The journalist spoke as if he was wanting to set a horribly crooked record straight, to defend Doris from a calumny that would now surely follow her in death as it had in life. Was that slur against women, against Doris, the heartless, 'unnatural woman', what the journalist feared as the news of her death turned into a week or so of obituaries, certainly praising but never leaving out the two abandoned children a continent away? Would it now be set in concrete? As I recall, although the subject had been broached by interviewers, at lunches, dinners, in telephone calls, and Doris was asked about how she felt now about having left her two oldest children (ten and eight), no battle raged between the pro- and anti-factions when it came to the matter of Doris 'walking out' on her children.

Nothing like the fuss, say, about Martin Amis's teeth. When it came up, her lips thinned and stiffened, she closed her eyes for a fraction of a second longer than was required for a mere blink, and a deep drawing in of the breath signalled the effort involved in having to experience the tedium of that question again. If you need help visualising it, imagine the present monarch's face at having come, toe to excrement, upon a steaming pile of dog shit while taking one of her favourite walks. I don't have favourite walks (or even like walking), but Doris did. Queen Mary's Gardens was one of them. I imagine the Queen having favourite walks, too. Doris always waved the question of Jean and John away and the subject was changed. How? I'm really not sure. I suspect it was partly that withering look she used to keep predators at bay, especially that trick of closing her eyes just a little longer than necessary, and also the simple fact that she never, with few exceptions, cared what people thought about her.

When my first novel was published in 1986, a journalist called to do an interview. I vaguely remembered him from a party at someone's house and arranged to meet him at a nearby coffee shop. My first novel revolved around a couple engaged in S&M sex and the interviewer immediately asked me about the details of my sex life. I said I didn't want to discuss it. He smiled, knowing about print-innocent sprats like me. It's like this, he said, showing me the ropes: you discuss it with me, I write it up the way you want it and it will keep the other journalists away. And, moreover, if I told my story to him, I wouldn't have some of the slimier papers making things up. I would be in control of what people thought of me. He spoke meticulously, treading the line between bully and guardian angel. I was impressed with his technique, but very far from persuaded. I said I didn't have anything of any interest to say. But, he said, now moving in with the big weapon, you can have a real influence on what people think of you. Again I doffed my cap at Doris, her withering looks and shrugs. 'But,' I said, 'you don't see; I don't care what people think of me, even if there was anything to think.' I checked myself up and down, a quick but thorough examination, and found nothing quaking or solid matter liquidising, not even the hint of a headache, not the slightest desire for drugs or other chemicals that would assuage the terror that I really didn't have about anything. I'm sorry, Sid, I said, but I don't give a toss what anyone who I don't know thinks of me. I don't even care what those who do know me think. Frankly, Sid – I took a deep breath to hold the moment – frankly, my dear, I don't give a damn. Sid left his half-cold coffee and the unpaid bill. 'You'll be sorry. Everyone cares. In the end everyone cares.' And off went Rhett or Scarlett (depending on how you'd like to allegorise), leaving me and my dirty washing in a rare state of tranquillity. It turned out that I really didn't care. And I doubted that anyone who didn't know me was likely to care what I might have been up to. I'd have to be much further up the tree of fame than I intended to climb to become interesting. A lesson I certainly learned in part from Doris.

I've never had the sense that a great wrong had been done to Doris in the vicious world of literary dinner parties. I heard no gossip to speak of, but it is a little strange, actually, that no tabloid story emerged at any point. It might have been because I was too close to catch the whispers, indoors rather than out there, or that the whispers stopped when I came within hearing distance. I suppose I was seen as too close now to the subject not to be considered a danger. What surprises me, given that her life in her twenties through to her forties encompassed several of the touchiest aspects of some of the touchiest subjects in social discourse – motherhood, the parental division of labour, sex roles, gender identity, the family and its constitution, ambitious women, sexually active women and so on – is that no one much cared. Lots of good books, a Nobel, a lively though not notorious sex life. Not much there for an obituary, except to talk mostly about the writing. A situation which would have pleased Doris very much. And really no one cares much about books. Football, yes, tennis, yes, the corruption of the very rich, yes, a bit. But, novels, writing? That shrug. Doris who? 'Oh, the Nobel Prize, was it? Oh, I thought it was for physics and that. Did she win the Booker?'

To me, the most interesting aspect of Doris arriving in London with her third child and a novel, while her other two children remained with their father, was that it required a move across the world. It was, as I see it, an instance of Doris putting as much space between herself and an unwelcome truth as she could. From the way she described Southern Rhodesia, I thought, as she did, that she couldn't possibly stay if she was to do what she wanted to do. To any questions (not many, I'd got the message) about leaving the children, it was clear that living alone in London with three children under ten was all but impossible. I am a feminist and a mother. I applaud the escape to freedom of a woman living her own life at such a time and in such a place, and her determination to fulfil her passion, to experience the power of her need to write.

The backwoods town of Salisbury may have seen a little excitement during the war, with passing armies, and loud meetings of brothers and sisters of the left arguing their position on this and that, but once the war was over and the soldiers on R&R had gone back to their real homes, it became a desert for a young woman looking for her place in the world. I get the need to flee, but no matter how I try to put myself in her place, I am perplexed by her emotional ability actually to do it. I'm struck most of all by her finding a way to justify taking the one child and leaving the others. Perhaps it was simple common sense – a phrase she often used. She did tell me that she was sure Jean and John would be well looked after by the Wisdoms, but thought that Gottfried was too immersed in his politics to take much notice of Peter. (Gottfried died, an ambassador for East Germany, in an ambush in Uganda in 1979.) She showed both her immense personal bravery and her ruthlessness in support of her cause. She was perfectly right that her project – of being a known and admired writer beyond Salisbury – required that she leave the provinces of southern Africa. I suppose it would have been possible to write, a white woman living in Africa (as it was for Nadine Gordimer), nearer to her two first children, but it would have meant giving up a world of experience denied to her in post-war Salisbury (not having rid itself of apartheid), with its frozen middle-class attitudes to women – what they could do, and how they could do it. She wanted to be recognised as the writer she was, not as the scandalous woman who dared to write novels certain to be banned: surely what would have happened to any of the first few books she would write, *The Grass Is Singing* especially, in which a woman stranded on an island of boredom and igno-rance does her worst to the gin-drinking English émigrés and takes a black servant for her lover. Real writers (as opposed to crowd-pleasers) are often uncomfortable if they aren't writing on the edge and even crossing it, rather than policing their prose to keep away the censors – particularly that inner one.

Once she had left, she was put on the prohibited immigrants list and banned from re-entering Rhodesia, until independence in 1979. Then she did go back to Zimbabwe, though only occasionally, and saw John and Jean, by then in their thirties and forties. She spoke publicly of the tedium of motherhood: 'No one can write with a child around,' she once pronounced ('pronounced' is a word I try to avoid in introducing recorded speech, but here and with other quotes from Doris it is apt). 'It's no good. You just get cross.' 'I'm very proud of myself that I had the guts to do it,' she told Barbara Ellen of the *Observer* in 2001. 'I've always said that if I hadn't left that life, if I hadn't escaped from the intolerable boredom of colonial circles, I'd have cracked up, become an alcoholic. And I'm glad that I had the bloody common sense to see that.' Common sense, again. There was usually comedy lurking in it somewhere. I remember Doris ringing while Roger and I were in the middle of a furious argument about the details of how the two of us would split up our treasures. House, child, hi-fi. It was clear from my voice that something was up, so I told her what she had unwittingly parachuted into. 'Oh, for heaven's sake,' she said, 'do give all that emotional nonsense a rest. Come round and have a cup of tea and we can talk sensibly about it.' I put the phone down and before I'd finished my sentence telling Roger what Doris had said, we were both laughing helplessly in recognition of the simplicity with which Doris approached little matters like leaving a husband or wife and sorting out the children. Just stop being emotional. How? We were upset.

Old friends. Best friends. Had a child. Had changed feelings towards each other. Was love in its degrees to be recognised? Oh, just stop it. Have a cup of tea. Use your common sense. What is all this nonsense about periods of adjustment, unequal feelings? Just be sensible. There is a Sufi story she was fond of that had the Charlie Chaplinesque figure of the Mullah Nasruddin in the middle of the night going round and round a lamp post on his knees. Asked what he was doing, he said he was looking for his keys. Where did you drop them? Oh, over there, the mullah says, indicating a spot a good distance away. So why are you looking for them here? There's more light here, says the mullah. Neither Roger nor I found the mullah helpful in our real-life crisis, and he didn't solve the problem when the drum we'd schlepped back from Morocco in our Morris 1000 had to be divvied up, but out he came anyway, along with the biscuits.

Oh, Doris would say to anyone in any kind of emotional trouble, why can't people just be sensible? Once or twice I shouted back: because we're people. The answer carried no weight at all. If we insisted on behaving like idiots what did we expect? The answer was clear: there was no hope of ever being right as Doris was right. Those furious footsteps as I walked from the bus to Kingscroft Road snapped to the rhythm of Doris's certainty. Not just that she was right, but that to be right, like her, was simple; to have the emotional control she had was just a matter of pulling oneself together, of not being 'ridiculous'. And it was true that the argument stopped for the time being, even if the details of the argument remained unresolved. Sometimes being sensible meant burying your head in the sand, or saying goodbye to old friends who didn't agree with you. Or maybe 'sensible' is one of those words that mean different things to different people.

She often spoke of missing Africa, with a lyricism about the landscape, the skies, the veldt, the sunrise, the animals, the smell after rain. She never mentioned people, or only in groups, overheard singing and dancing. It wasn't racism, but part of her picture of the place she loved and missed. It always sends a chill down my spine (as it did hers) to think of those deprived, deracinated people being given work looking after other people's children, hundreds of miles away from their own families.

She insisted she was still a farm girl at heart, hunting small game, defying the nuns who taught her nothing useful, never taking much interest in style or fashion. I'm sure she would have brought Africa along with her if she could have, but nothing was going to keep her there if it wasn't going to be the Africa she wanted. And it certainly wasn't socially or politically. But she took Peter with her to London. Like a mascot? As if taking one child would make up for leaving two? I don't know. When the subject was brought up it was always a matter of female freedom, by which she meant her freedom primarily, and how the life she was leading would have stifled the writer in her. She had been a tomboy who wanted to hang on to the privileges that boys and men had. In a way, she reminded me of Margaret Thatcher, who was hailed by many feminists as a blow struck for feminism and turned out to be nothing of the sort. Doris used her femininity where it was useful or enjoyable, but had no interest at all in the actual politics of feminism, or in changing the economic and social position of women except for the particular purpose of giving women the choice to leave their families. Or, in the case of the Africa she had known, giving women the choice to stay and look after their own families.

I remember a row she had one lunchtime with an American lesbian couple, about a woman in similar social and financial circumstances to Doris's before she left Frank Wisdom. The visitors were wondering why on earth the woman didn't just up and leave. Doris had, after all. Eventually she exploded, talking to the women as if they were children who knew nothing about the world and its difficulties. She spoke as she gathered and clattered plates and made her way to the kitchen, where the last word was kept. Her voice, harsh, barely controlled, told you she had now lost patience with you and your ignorance. 'You can't just up and leave when you've got a house and two children and no money of your own. How stupid can you people get? Most people aren't rich and privileged like you.' Unhappy women were all over the place, stuck in suburbias all over the world; but they couldn't just leave, with nowhere to go, no money, no support. The women were silenced. Doris took a moment in the kitchen preparing the pudding and rearranging her furious expression. When she returned to the living room no one mentioned the subject of women leaving their unsatisfactory men, or the fact that Doris's argument, if that was what it was, was made without any reference to her own very real experience.

Outbursts of this kind (not all of them shouted) were generally known to those of us who were close to her as 'being told off by Doris'. They were received in silence, no one took or was invited to take a different position. They silenced the company, who quickly started talking about something else. Asked what I thought about her novel *Love, Again*, I said I found it improbable, given that it was posing as a realistic novel, that the man and woman who had fallen in love in middle age refused to have sex with each other because each had a husband or wife they didn't love but who needed them in some way. I wasn't arguing that they should leave their spouses, but that their affair should have continued through the years unconsummated suggested an unnecessary sort of morality in a modern, grown-up, realist setting. Doris gave me one of her looks. The several other people in the room hushed their conversation. 'Well, it's a good thing, Jenny, that there are some people still left who, unlike you, take sex seriously.' Again, Doris hoisted herself up from the carpet in mid-sentence, and went to fetch another plate of biscuits.

With increasing impatience over the years, Doris rejected the idea that *The Golden Notebook* was intended to be a work of feminism. It's hard to see why, unless she wanted to make the point that writing of any kind is always a private, autobiographical affair even if it isn't only that. By the end of her thinking life she got very angry at the suggestion that she was a feminist icon. In the 1990s and later, she was writing and talking about the damage that 'radical' feminism was doing to the spirit of men who were becoming wimps as a result. In that interview in 2001 with Barbara Ellen, she is quoted as saying: 'It's become absolutely automatic. If it was some polemical crusade, it might be something, but it's like young women have got ten minutes to spare, so they may as well spend it rubbishing men. It's part of the culture now. There's an unconscious bias in our society: girls are wonderful; boys are terrible. And to be a boy, or young man, growing up, having to listen to all this, it must be painful.' And here, I suspect, was another reason Peter was as he was that had nothing to do with Doris's parenting skills.

Many of her later books (for example, *The Marriages Between Zones Three, Four and Five*; *The Making of the Representative of Planet Eight*; *The Cleft*) are hymns to atavistic battles; they describe trysts between men and women experiencing uncommon ecstasies of love and necessary separations, all unsullied by picking children up from school, or paying the gas bill late. Women with flowing hair familiar from Middle Earth and suchlike fantasy fiction are followed by white horses whose manes they stroke and into whose ears they whisper. *The Cleft* is actually a prehistoric tale of the muscularity of women discovering their creative reproductive powers while the men break away to make discoveries and have adventures by sea and on foot.

Doris wrote to John and Jean, and they came to London to visit as children a few times. Jean came for a couple of months when she was in her late teens or early twenties, and I was living in Charrington Street. Like many other visitors who came from all over the world to sit at Doris's feet and gather wisdom (in Jean's case, a late-flowering mother/daughter relationship), she was given to me to take care of because Doris was in the middle of an especially difficult bit in the current book. 'Take her shopping. Show her around. Let her meet your friends,' were her instructions. But our worlds were so different, Jean's and mine, and so unimaginable each to the other, that the visit could only cause pain, and I think perhaps was intended to. This was a thing about Doris: it was never clear whether she knew how painful or disastrous her actions or pronouncements could be.

Was it just carelessness, a desperation to get back to her typewriter, or did she know perfectly well the anguish she would cause these former fans or relatives?

Jean and I went wandering around the centre of what was thought of as London in full swing. We visited boutiques, where Jean tried on clothes she couldn't imagine wearing at home, and bookshops whose books would not get through customs; she sat in an agony of shyness in the pub with old men and drunk poets. I recently had an email from someone who remembers Doris 'trying to palm off ' a young woman 'barely out of her teens' on him at a party, and the excruciating embarrassment the girl showed at the whole incident. He wondered in his email whether it had been me. I don't remember, but I'm fairly sure it was Jean, very far from being comfortable with casual meetings and beddings with strangers.

Wilfulness? The necessity of art? The pain that others have to tolerate so that art could be made? I don't know. I know about feeling trapped and that sometimes you have to be somewhere else in order to do what you need to do, but I couldn't imagine leaving my daughter Chloe permanently in order to fulfil my promise. Perhaps that's just cowardice and Doris would say, I think, that I was lucky I didn't have to. I was in the privileged position of having enough money to live on from teaching, and then when I had a breakdown and actually started to write my first novel she gave me an allowance. And I had a husband committed to our daughter and to sharing the childcare. I hadn't grown up in the boondocks, where one wrong footfall caused an avalanche of disapproval. For all the misogyny that exists even now, as bad and perhaps worse than in my childhood, I never felt that I was held back by being a woman. But I knew that others were. In any case, she wasn't alone; she had support from friends and comrades, and from Joan Rodker, whose flat at the top of her house Doris rented. And there was Peter, there was always and would always be Peter, the chosen one; Peter would be there for Doris and he would certainly be there for the Wisdom children who had been left behind. There is a cruelty there (is it possible that it was 'just' thoughtlessness?). There is self-justification that can make some sense to one's own conscience. But it's very hard to buy once you put Peter into the equation, and then on top of that add me, both of us at the high point of adolescence. I think I know something of the power of the necessity to write, and the importance of finding a place to do so. But however highly you value Doris's wisdom in her books, what is happening here? I can't speak of the two older children and the ways in which they managed to cope with their abandonment, but at Doris's funeral, Jean (John having died of a heart attack) stood and spoke of being glad that Doris had left her and let her (Jean) have a life of her own.

It was something that Peter never had. Peter had no life of his own, ever. No life at all, except perhaps an exotic inner life. And I have doubts even about that. He and I didn't like each other from the start, but even though we didn't have a good relationship, we were engaged in each other's lives for much of our own. He had the self-important but kindly thought of helping me out when he heard of my troubles. He was sixteen. There wasn't much chance of his understanding how dangerous or painful this was for him to do. Peter's existence was the saddest and emptiest I can imagine. His funeral gave those of us choosing its form a problem. What kind of eulogy could be written for a man who from nineteen had never worked or had a proper job, no real relationships, sexual or otherwise, who had barely gone outside for the last half of his life, who lived alone with his mother, lay on his bed when he wasn't watching television in the afternoon and evening and eventually became so gross, in the sense of fat and uncouth, that very few people could put up with it? How much he knew of how the world saw him is another mystery. It seemed that his life had effectively stopped at around nineteen, but then we found a drawing done by a friend of ours from school at around that age which showed a strikingly good-looking young man, smoking a cigarette with his head lolling back, as if waiting for us all to come and find him his place in the world. But it was there, in the inviting drawing, full of confidence and promise, that Peter's world came to a stop. His friends from St Christopher's came and we remembered the fun we sometimes had at Charrington Street, sitting around the kitchen table, or gathered up in Peter's room. While I listened on my Dansette to Bob Dylan's first album (1962 – with Doris, along with a million other parents or surrogate parents, bellowing from down-stairs: 'Turn that noise off. He can't even sing!'), Peter was grabbed by the surreal, and the big, emotional choral anthems. We talked to people who knew and remembered those days, hard as it was.

His funeral included the Goons's song, 'Ying Tong Idlle I Po', which he used to sing far too often; there was a reading about Eeyore being stuck in the river expressing his deep conviction that no one would rescue him; the Red Army Choir singing 'Kalinka' was another song Peter belted out and sang along with during the holidays; another A. A. Milne, this time written for Winnie-the-Pooh, 'The More It Snows (Tiddely-Pom)'; and finally, Blake's 'Jerusalem', the music by Hubert Parry, and sung at the end of every school year at St Chris with unthinking gusto. The old days. People left smiling. I couldn't have imagined it possible when we started to plan it. But there was nothing I knew of any evident pleasure or fun later than the early 1970s. After that he was more or less a prisoner, aiding and abetting his warden in a world that grew smaller and smaller. When you tried to describe it, people narrowed their eyes in disbelief, trying to imagine the life I was clearly exaggerating; no one could live such a non-eventful existence for decades, let alone someone with so many advantages. Peter's life, to people who were not familiar with it, was a made-up tale; an impossibility. That's not to say that things didn't sometimes happen to Peter, at least in those youthful days when generosity, solemnity and thoughtlessness could go hand in hand.

One thing that happened was me. If there is only so much social energy to go round in any given group, you could say that I elbowed in, loud, loving argument and discussion, and took Peter's portion. Being there was my good fortune, perhaps, but I also know how hard it was to extract oneself from Doris once she had decided you were 'one of hers'. Peter wrote a letter that allowed a voluble teenage girl into his house, to live with his mother while he was away at boarding school. It might have been some kind of gift (conscious or unconscious) to his mother, or a way of telling her that he needed more or less from her, or better attention. Years later, a friend told me that in the past Peter had said to him that 'the worst thing that could happen to me would be if Jenny became a successful novelist'. It wasn't my fault that I was, as papers and magazines have suggested, a cuckoo in Peter's nest. I know that I was, even if I was not directly responsible. But that became one of the stories explaining Peter's 'oddness'. Journalists came up to me at parties, sometimes when Doris was there too, to check whether what Doris had just (or recently) told them was true, that Peter's life was ruined and he was made sick by my going to live with them, and taking his space in the household. I had no way of denying it. It's very possible that I helped sink Peter, by taking his place in 'his' house and by getting on with a regular sort of life. I was Peter's shadow, as Doris and, I suppose, Peter saw it, who had taken his place in the light. So I just replied: 'If she says so.'

Still, few people could believe that a person of sixteen could have his life ruined that way, without there being something else that had been going on for much longer to cause what almost seemed a lifelong catatonia. I didn't swallow Doris's story. But I didn't deny it, and I didn't ask Doris why she was saying these things to journalists at parties. Healthy people don't lie down in the middle of the road and allow a bus to roll over them – not unless something in them is acting out damage done long before. I was not a gift from Peter to his mother, but a curse. I could see that. Peter had perhaps despaired of Doris giving him what he needed, even if he didn't know exactly what that was. I was a gesture, a question, a conversation he wasn't able to start with Doris. Perhaps, without mentioning the children back in Africa, he had tried to rebalance the family. Or he was hoping to deflect something on to me. Or he was just having a kind moment and didn't think hard enough about the possible consequences. I was a disaster for both of them. Doris, however, was forty-four when she got Peter's letter and wrote to me. Another generous act. A kindness almost beyond measure. And she added to it by telling me that there was no need to be grateful. Someone had helped her, I would help someone . . . But she was a grown woman, taking on damaged goods that Dr Watt had warned her about. I don't know what, if any, precautions she took; essentially I think she thought she could manage without them. What was Doris thinking of? As the beneficiary of all this kindness, and as a person now in my late sixties, I believe Doris took a grave risk with three people's lives, and I can't really untangle the strands that might tell me why.

Almost every day since I began writing about my cancer I have received a letter or an email from someone who has read or remembered and liked my work; they talk about the recent pieces about my cancer or my memories of my teenage years and my relationship with Doris Lessing, my older books, fiction and non-fiction, something they've read or remembered. They're remarkably kind (my paranoia wonders, but I fight back the idea that the *London Review of Books*'s editors hold on to the ones that are not so positive). They are well meant, offering as solace the people 'out there' in the real world who have enjoyed my work, and they hope that I will be well and that I will continue writing. One or two suggest I prostrate myself (an inevitable image here of Audrey Hepburn face down in the stone-paved aisle) and pray to the Holy Mother of Jesus, who will cure anyone who asks and believes in her. Even a Jew? Why? A gratuity. A gift given freely, regardless. And yet Mary

Mother of Christ doesn't really give freely – she wants you to ask and for you to believe in her. Not quite gratuitous. Others offer pills or potions that the medical establishment has overlooked, but which in the right doses (always either huge or minute) are KNOWN to cure all kinds of cancer, as attested by people whose lives have been saved by enough fresh carrot juice to sink a submarine. There aren't any negative or abusive messages. That rather alarms me. I'd be sick to death of me by now. The weird medicines are all offered with the best of intentions, though best of all are emails that simply say: 'No need to write back, I just want to say I hope you stay well as long as you can, and that your writing has meant a lot to me.' Of course I reply and say thank you as often as I can, because I'm genuinely grateful to receive such messages from strangers.

But, in all honesty (which always seems to trump good manners), I'm not genuinely grateful at all. Not in that dark place where I am a naughty, angry child. I can't feel genuinely anything much because that train left the platform before I knew it was there, or I slept, as it stopped then started off again without a thought for its sleepy passenger. There is supposed to be a psychological state at which we all have to arrive and where we rest or make a final effort before we can receive our certificate for having done right. Perhaps I *was* asleep when the shards of glass dropped from the playful cherubims' hands and fell arbitrarily into the eyes or hearts of some, but only some. Broken mirrors falling through the sky, to change the hearts and minds of a few people so that they can see only the bleak side of anything good or innocuous. I really can't get away without finding myself in the fairy or hobgoblin stories. That must be my sliver of looking glass, reflecting a place where everything is not what it seems, a world of my own making, of tickling death and then hiding between my own legs, as one hid behind one's mother's in shame or anxiety. Goblin. Hobgoblin. There once was an ugly duckling. *There* was a promise for those who saw the world as it really was. But promises aren't always kept and I can't tolerate unfulfilled promises. My head is full of dark, terrorising tales, you will have noticed. Collected or made up on the spot. Can there be any more stories left? Always, into perpetuity. The stories never run out, especially the 'real ones', the ones that actually happened and press forward impatiently awaiting their turn, like elephants' teeth. When the teeth run out – the ones planted before birth in the world – the elephant starves to death. The wicked cruelty of nature. Always another trick up its sleeve. Some of us will suffocate, some will starve. Some will spend their days waiting for the end of the story. I guess some people don't. Certainly, I doubt that elephants fret about the way the end will come.

And then, after the daily busyness of radiotherapy, there was nothing. Or at least it was amazing busyness for me, who can remain contentedly indoors, staring, for weeks on end. Now there was nothing else on the menu. Nothing new, anyway. Food still tasted foul and bitter, I was still tired enough to sleep an extra four hours a day. But the treatment was over. It would take three months to finish its work inside my body, then a scan to see if anything had happened. If the placebo effect works for one in three people (there's that ragged seaman again, his bird rotting, rotting, rotting around his neck; why won't someone do something?), the odds were good for me, though better if I had received a non-placebo and perhaps I had. I just had to trust my luck. There's the problem. I don't trust anyone, not their shy words of good intent, not their commiserations, not their active and proven medication. I know too about the nocebo effect, where medically active drugs don't work on a third of patients who are told they are taking corn-flour. What could anyone give me that could definitively improve my health? And what is my health when most of the unwellness came from the treatment? I've got the place surrounded, Mr Earp. And there's only one piece of magic left if faith is left out. Love, there's love. But if I arrived on earth without a capacity for faith, when right now, with a death sentence tattooed on me, I simply can't find this faith they talk of, that easy answer to the terror of death and dying, how the hell am I going to place my trust in love, mine, his, the spirit of the planet? 'Whatever love means' to each entity that uses it, it's time they used it. Or teach me how. See, as soon as you slide off towards the easy answer – trust in me – you start to sound like a feeble-minded prince with nothing to do. Anyway, it's a little late at sixty-eight. Quality of life. Well, of course there is. But right now I can't see them holding me down like ballast. I could even take a small lie or two at the moment.

I've got no apparatus to throw over myself as I make the swan dive. I'm just out there, alone without even anyone to lie the truth to me. Carried on the wind, swinging on a breeze, but entirely alone.

So after nearly a year (let's leave be the six months of depression and the changing of medications before the machine checking on the pulmonary fibrosis also found, by accident, a tumour in my lung), after this boxing match of a year, Onc Doc was able to tell me that his chemo treatment had at least stopped the growth and movement of the lung cancer ('Though we

can't know for how long'), while the lifetime's allowance of radiation had greatly worsened the fibrosis. It
would now most likely be the fibrosis – for which there
is no cure, only a slowing of progression – that would
kill me.

For how long? This uncertainty is difficult. Perhaps
a year, the younger, more relaxed Doctor Fibes told
me. But then that caution: of course we can't be sure.
I might get an infection; just a minor thing without a
properly functioning immune system could escalate into
pneumonia. More deadly. Of course they can't, they're
working with statistics taken from studies made years
and worlds apart. We're back to square one. Everyone
is different, we can't make that kind of judgement.
The answer is – with the new drugs, if they work on
me – 'perhaps a year'. But then again . . . I've never been
really ill, apart from those sweaty children's infections
it's best to get over and done with. I don't exactly feel ill
now. I'm trapped in a mesh of steroid effects. I've been
put on them to stall the damage done by not having used
steroids with the radiotherapy. They may slow down the
infections, but have hideous side-effects; within three
weeks of taking a 'very moderate dose, of the weakest
steroid they make', my weight had shot from eight stone
to eleven stone. Fat that feels as if my body has been
stuffed with some alien gel settled in particular places.
My face and body have rounded. Cushing's syndrome.
The shock I get from an ill-advised glance into a looking glass trembles down my spine. No one has ever seen
me fat before. But it's necessary and the doctors don't
consider fatness important compared to three months'
more life. This is because they are men in suits or neat
women who have not taken steroids themselves. It's like
a punishment. But for what?

In addition, the steroids, or something else, keep making me totter and fall, at home, in the street, so I can't get beyond my front door without someone to help me along. Every sitting down and standing up is fraught with the danger of another fall and another break. The Poet (it's so good to call him by the name I gave him when nothing was wrong) has to help me dress and go up or down the stairs. It's about as tough on him as it is on me. I was fully of the opinion when the cancer diagnosis was first made that he had the worst of it, but since trying to haul myself up from the ground after getting out of a taxi – only after a few long minutes did the driver get out of his seat to help me up – my opinion is changing. I am the old lady falling down and lacking the muscle power to get up. One of the most humiliating conclusions you can come to about yourself: it won't get better (although the 'fatness' is water retention). But now, providing I don't look at myself in the mirror in the hall, I begin to see (as in *feel*) that it doesn't matter so much. As I write there is a world refugee crisis. I've never had to cope with that. That little cancer in my lung, and the growing forest of fibrotic alveoli will kill me, but something would have. Please, a real plea, not to speak to me, or anyone else, of 'bravery'. I need to be told the story in which it doesn't matter, a story of the millions who've died already. Of the millions who are to die and live in terrible conditions. And yet I still tell the doctor and hospice nurse both conversationally and on a signed living will that I want to die easily, not an agitated death. Imagine all those millions who have never been given that choice. Not that I suppose anyone but a masochist would choose the agitated death. Just enough of a coma so I can wave a weak goodbye and let them get on with their lives. That's hard enough to do. My God, people like me have been given lives and choices no other generation has ever had. I wonder why. I'm speaking, of course, of a white, Western cohort which the generations on either side quite rightly resent. What the hell did we do to deserve to have it so easy? Nothing. On one side the twentieth-century wars, then in gratitude free education, housing, a long state-funded playtime that went on into our thirties; then the next generation where it all has to be paid for. The vital welfare state that is concerned with hearts and minds rather than outcomes and value for money. But for fuck's sake, get it back, kids. Fight for what was our right. Get angry.

I am interested in understanding how it comes about that in spite of my upper body's intention to go one way, my legs go in quite another direction, so that I scuttle about trying to get both parts of my body to pay attention to each other. It's something like finding oneself on a frozen lake without skates or experience. Again the docs and nurses don't seem to address this new difficulty in my life. I ended up yelling 'Help!' the other day, stuck three stairs from the middle landing, when I knew the house to be empty. And it seems like the bad vibes are spreading. (How right to have had that cliché all the while for when no other cliché will do.) Almost everything I do goes wrong or is unsightly. (I was already assured that my hair wouldn't fall out, so there's that: Rapunzel, just on my way up. Oh, do stop moaning. If you don't let your hair down, what can I do?) My hands tremble, making me look as if I'm continually one over the eight. I feel I need an exquisite silver necklace with the words 'I'm not mad, I'm ill' engraved on one side, and 'Ouch!' on the other.

In other, practical ways, I've done it right. I thought of these monthly essays straight away. Who knows when they will finish, but in the meantime they give me some thinking and writing to do. Enough, but not too much. Should I find myself hanging by my teeth I'll just declare the end the winner and bow out gratefully. If that pneumonia gets me unexpectedly, I'm sure someone will let you know. No hymns, please. Except, maybe Janis Joplin's 'Ball and Chain'.

The time I have left is roughly in sync with the original potshot. A year's treatment gives me between one and two years. And still I only feel deprived of not watching the grandchildren, two of them now, become their own people. For now, they remain delightful, a special medicine whose main side-effect is a painful sadness, the cure for which is to forget about the workings of time. For the rest, apart from occasional terror of extinction, it seems reasonable enough, if the contented coma I've been promised actually happens. The terror is not, of course, occasional and contentment doesn't come into it. Where am I going? Nobody knows. Can I come with you? Aye, bye and bye. There is a kind of excitement. This, that I've never done, already done but previously, in a different form, an absolute otherness, nothingness, knowinglessness. That everyone has done, will do, world without end. The ending, and the world going on, going about its daily business. A world without me. To have known but not have any apparatus to know with. The excitement of a newness that is as old as the hills. My turn.

And the terror. I'm reading accounts of undertakers, crematorium workers, seeing a counsellor once a week who has spent ten years working in a hospice getting people ready for death, not doing the other thing of helping to continue and improve their lives. Those few days I spent in the local hospice, really to give the Poet some respite, and a woman in a nearby room was crying out, calling without words, moaning in unending misery. 'What is the matter with her?' I meant apart from the obvious. The nurse was in my room taking my blood pressure. 'Oh,' she said calmly, 'she's not ready. She hasn't thought enough about it and now it's very hard for her.' That's how I imagined dying. Being ready or not. Between a trembling of horror, and the quiet of sufficiency. I wanted help with that. To deal with absence, the coming of nothing; it begins to make sense. But I'm haunted by the 1950s – I'm living then, which I hardly did – until I get into bed and sleep again. Is that the dead haunting the living, or the living haunting the dead? It's happened several times now, always getting time wrong, looking out for my mother (to hide or seek?), finding the Poet as ignorant as I am about where to find or hide from the dead. But at least he knows what day it is, or whether it's day or night. That's a comfort. But what clot-headed dreams I have. How inelegant, how miserably concealed. And how strange that they come with me for the rest of the day or night, live around my shoulder, like the disgusting foxes that rested around my mother's neck. The 1950s, just after a war had ended, the children of a new era, the children playing in the bomb sites of something that has never been imaginable. The Blitz, the sirens, the rubble. Born two years later and only a few bomb sites remaining. Thrilling for us, warnings about all sorts of things from our parents. We got the butter and the best of the rationed food, while we played and listened to their stories, too incredible to believe. Our children, at least in this country, with no tales of war to tell; only music and clothes. Infuriating and a blessing for our parents, who had experienced the abyss staring back at them. I suppose their memories must have hung around their necks like stinking albatrosses, only for their children to turn out themselves to be an abyss gazing back at the next generation. Is it catching? Whose 1950s was I living?

————

A long time ago I'd concluded that there was no point in my life if I wasn't to be a writer. 'The Point' was very important. It still is. All I can manage to say when I'm deep in my underground terrain is 'What's the point?' Only earning my living writing. I had the ridiculous, chaotic childhood and had grown up. Nearly twenty, yet I still wasn't a writer. Or nearly twenty, yet I still hadn't written anything. A few ghastly poems, bits and patches I'd banged out on my typewriter, as if having written the first paragraph, it would get on with it and write itself. Actually there's a little truth in that. But from a young girl on, writing and being a writer was the only way I could think of to be, the only way to balance the down side of the seesaw. Why the hell had I had those greedy, self-absorbed, terrifying parents if it wasn't to have something to write about? It wasn't exactly superstitious, nor overtly religious (now one and the same thing). It was a matter of what I had been given and why. What to do with it. That also sounds superstitious, so perhaps I thought that something out there was weighing and balancing. Weirdly it was also somewhat true. Looking back, I see a frantic childhood and young womanhood and then in my late thirties it was the time for the lion to bed down with the lamb. Inside me and in the world outside. How calm that sounds. Actually, it sounded more like: WHAT THE FUCK DID I HAVE TO HAVE ALL THAT SHIT FOR?

But also, and incoherently, why hadn't I had an interesting childhood? Essential for writing, surely. Come from somewhere else. A triple-A childhood that conformed. That surely was a writer's background. All the people I'd read, and the people around Doris's table, had travelled, or worked their way out of the working class to be passionate about . . . I wasn't even clear which class I belonged to. Not working class exactly. Certainly not middle class, because that was what my mother reached for so desperately. But I was convinced that those who wrote had had lives that could be written about, interesting lives. And I hadn't had an interesting life. Yet, at the same time, the only answer to the miserableness of most of my childhood was that I ought to be a writer. Long before I'd ever heard of Doris Lessing, Bourne and Hollingsworth, the bins, psychiatric units, borderline personality disorder (and I never have found out whether it was the personality that was disordered or a crack in the wall of personality that threatened to flood my self into nowhere if I didn't keep a hold on it. I think that BPD was really a diagnosis meaning a young woman who didn't do as she was told and they didn't know how to deal with it). Anyway, before all that stuff, I'd wanted to be a writer. I think a journalist, because it was exciting and you only had to describe what was happening. I told myself stories, but I never wanted to write them down. They were like computer games for me to act out all the characters. Later it was a novelist, when I realised that novelists lived exactly as I wanted to live. At home, with a couch to sleep on when I lost the thread, and a beloved typewriter. Lunches and literary parties, not so much. Fame? Maybe. My finished book in its jacket in a bookshop window. Yes, but something told me it wasn't a satisfaction that would last for long. One look, pleasure and then Oh Christ, what about the next book? Or most simply a writer alone in a room and a couple of inches of typescript. Looking at it, half-done, two-thirds finished. I did that. Lying on the couch with a cigarette and half closing my eyes to see enough of the manuscript waiting to grow.

What actually happened was two or three years of London at the peak of the 1960s, living in Covent Garden when it was still a fruit and veg market, open all night, the sweet, rotting smell of damp fresh greens coming up to the flat where I lived above the grocer's stall down at street level. Get a cup of tea and a chat any hour of the day or night from the van down the road, and all the drugs you could keep in a large jar of jelly beans. We smoked hash all day and into the night, injected methedrine, which was wonderful until you started to come down and discovered a side of depression darker than you'd ever dreamed of. We listened to Bob Dylan and the Velvets, wandered into each other's rooms and beds, reading ancient texts, sharing joints and the latest weird science fiction. There simply wasn't time enough to get to the end of a sentence by Henry James. We lived on allowances from our parents, or in my case, from my saviour (she didn't see me any more, because I was a lost cause, but the allowance continued), and also on state unemployment benefit, or sickness benefit. It was so easy to be a layabout and read Sartre, it was as if they *wanted* us to do it. All the while they shouted at us, how we looked, the dangerous things we did, locking some of us up in prison, but it was as if the older generation were playing its part with less conviction. With one hand they threatened to send us to bed without any supper, while with the other they gave us the wherewithal to live the life we were leading. We, our generation, were playing cops and robbers. We read the Mahabharata, let in a little light pulp to our druggy lives. Word went out, the fuzz were busting in Covent Garden. All the drugs went down the loo and someone took charge of the hoover to get rid of bits of hash on the floor. Kids playing games. Except that some went to prison for a year or two. Not me. Then the methedrine got to be too much. I had to stop it, and while I was at it I might as well cut out the acid and barbiturates, all of it. Cleaning out the old cupboard, with all its bottles and boxes years out of date.

Somewhere in all this time, that is, from leaving Doris's in 1966 – or 1967 or thereabouts – and 1971 (my timing is extremely approximate, though not as approximate as it would be if you were to ask where I was this time last week), somewhere in that time I spent about four months in the North Wing of St Pancras Hospital, the psychiatric ward that took in all the emergency crazies and found them somewhere they could be treated for whatever ailed them. One side of the hospital was being given a lick of paint and it was officially announced that patients could make free with filthy walls and large tubs of paint while the other side of the unit was being fitted out. Art therapy didn't take. The walls remained filthy and colourless except for the lintel over a door from the large patients' sitting room into a small side room, where someone had written in dripping blood-red 'Abandon Hope All Ye Who Enter Her [*sic*]'. Then chaos. I wrote a story about the haunted other side of the hospital. Who can tell the painters from the patients?

It was here that I was put into a barbiturate sleep and then had to be hauled out of it when they discovered that

I was getting barbiturate poisoning. It was also where I met my friend Mr Amnesiac, a middle-aged man who had lost all his life except the present, but they found out his name, and that he'd left his house somewhere up north with a large chunk of cash to pay the rent and was found wandering in King's Cross Station, where he ended up in the unknown strays department with no money. His wife and daughter came to visit him. He didn't remember them at first but said they seemed very nice. So I found myself dumped by a man for his wife. The other result was that he became the amnesiac professor in *Briefing for a Descent into Hell* (a novel by Doris) with whom the Olympian gods toyed; he became Doris's seafarer endlessly at sea. There was a young girl in the hospital he was taken to. She stood out because she didn't wear knickers under her short, short skirt (remember, nothing new under the sun). Doris gave me a copy of the book and said she hoped I didn't mind her using 'my' character like that. I said no, but I could imagine writing about him myself, if I ever became a writer. I suppose the fact that she got on with it made the story hers in some way.

A couple of weeks ago, my nice hairdresser down the road had washed and dried my hair, and I went out the back way, where the Poet would pick me up and take me home – a couple of hundred yards back up the street, but I was too wobbly and wary to do it on foot, alone. Suddenly, while waiting for the Poet to arrive, my legs behaved impossibly and I crashed face down and lay in the concrete and gravel knowing that my forehead had been really cracked. I wondered if I was dead, and then decided that if I was wondering I was probably still alive. So after a moment resting with my face in the gravel, I shouted 'Help! Help!' at the top of my voice. Luckily the Poet drove up, saw me lying face down and managed not to run me over. It turned out my bellowing for help was about loud enough for a passing ant to hear. The Poet got me into the car and off we went to spend the next eight hours in A&E. The next morning I had a stitch in my forehead where the gravel had made a size-able hole, and two enormous black eyes, like the mask of Zorro. 'Can you count back from twenty to one?' the student doc asked, checking whether I had damaged my brain. I said 'Yes', which I thought should be enough to put an end to this affair. But she insisted that I go through the whole rigmarole. I may have sung it, just to keep it interesting. To say that the side-effects from my meds have let me down would be the worst ever joke. But the hell with it. My legs let me down. So here I still am starting the next week with just the one stitch, a bump the size of a pigeon's egg, a deep hole in my fore-head and a pair of black eyes which in the right light look like water spilled over petrol. And my wrist is all shaken up, the same wrist I broke last time. Oh well. Worst, my clean hair was caked with blood.

And now the new pills have arrived, delivered myste-riously by a courier in a van because they've been passed by Nice for hospital use but not for GPs or pharmacists. It takes three weeks to get up to my full dose while the steroids go down at the same rate. *O the mind, mind has mountains; cliffs of fall* . . . Still, in a few weeks I will be off the steroids, which made me a balloon that the Poet had to hold on to to stop me floating away. Not that I'm in a very floaty form in my present state. Will I get back to a proper weight? I have to eat lunch, so I can have the pills three times a day, which is not my idea of a proper life. I'm a snacker. And no grapefruit. Normally

I wouldn't give grapefruit a second glance, but I feel the desire coming on. I think I've done something to my left knee because I can't put any weight on that leg without wailing, but the nice doctor prodded and pushed, and deduced from the 'ow's and 'aie's that it was probably just bruised. I'm back to taking the stairs one at a time. Blessed grandson and tiny granddaughter came on Sunday. 'Granjen, why are you so slow?' 'All the better to . . . ' Oh, I am so sad not to be seeing more of their growing up.

The harmless quietness of the time after drugs, sex and rock, when I was teaching wayward children, interrupted the narrative. I lived in bedsitters and hospitals for the year or so after my spell in the North Wing. I can't understand it. Just the thought of some of the places I lived and worked and shivered in makes me tremble with depression, but I was young. Eventually they had a bed for me at the Maudsley, where I settled in nicely for nine months. My best friend (whom I didn't yet know) was waiting for me (whom she didn't yet know) with a virgin game of Scrabble, set out on the table between her and the empty chair she was waiting for someone to sit on. I sat on it immediately. We played pathological games of Scrabble. She was mad as a rat, but she says it was me who was mad. Well. She has become a poet and I've become me. The Maudsley our alma mater. We were very bad girls, in the very bad girls' side of the ward. At the other end, the good girls resided. They played Cliff Richard and one actually announced herself cured of an inability to walk without lurching from one side of the street to the other by going to the Billy Graham razzamatazz and his putting his hands on her. Ach, Billy Graham where are you when you're needed? We took Cliff off the record player and put Hendrix on. It's funny how things fall out.

As for heartache, we – S, let's say, and me – took turns and looked after each other. When there was a hump in the bed under which a poor girl lay, we (she or I) sat at the end of the bed protecting her (or me) from the nurses, shouting: 'Come on, get out of bed.' There was a gentle kindness and fierce craziness in Ward 6. I want to write an opera about it, S and I working together (most of our recollections are very similar), but we won't. The heartache passed, but we knew it was there. We got heartache holidays. When I cut myself, S came with me across the road to King's College Hospital, to make sure I was being treated properly. Hopeless, as it turned out: as soon as she saw blood dripping from my wrist, she fainted and they thought she was the patient. They put sticks in her mouth to stop her from biting her tongue, while I shouted that she had just fainted and if she woke up strapped to a stretcher, she would really go off her head. I waved my bloody-razored arm at them to show what the situation was. In any other generation this would all have been strange. It wasn't strange to us. Funny, sometimes, but not strange.

When Doris met with my consultant he told her that my depression was due to my not being in a real relation with her, and that I felt I couldn't behave the way most adolescents behaved with their real family, knowing there would always be a reprieve. Doris returned fuming and told me this, finishing: 'You don't feel you can't say anything because you're not my real daughter, do you?' The double bind was familiar to me from reading R. D. Laing and others, so I sat on the edge of my bed and said 'No', as insincerely as I could manage. 'Of course not,' Doris said, 'the man's an idiot.' We – that is, Doris – had reached the end of the 'psychology is everything' phase, as Sufism arrived and seemed to her to lock all her former passions together, neat and tight as a Rubik's Cube.

The vile mustard-coloured coat, my first 'grown-up' item of clothing, hung in the airing cupboard alongside some marijuana that Doris had grown in the garden her first summer in the house and was now drying out; I never wore the coat again, though we did smoke the dope. Being grown up and behaving like a lady were the main words of advice my mother had had for me on the way from Brighton. Not such bad advice from someone for whom every new meeting held the possibility of 'getting somewhere'. A marriage proposal – for her or me, it didn't matter. A fairy-like personage would recognise the dreadful way life had treated her, and make recompense with an elegant flat and a fistful of paper money, or a pot of gold. 'Behaving like a lady' somehow cleaned the stained glass.

There was one photo, among the many in the large cardboard box my mother gave to Bill, the boilerman, in the hope that one day, after we'd been evicted and found ourselves in a grand mansion, she'd get it back, one photo that I looked at with wonder. My mother was sitting on some steps down to the sea in Monte Carlo or somewhere in the south of France. Walking down those steps to the sea was a man I'd only heard of from her. It was Douglas Fairbanks, Jr. A playboy who lived in a mansion and played as boys with rich mothers and

fathers do. My mother was posing, with one leg pointing downwards to the sea and the other playfully curled
beneath her in her white playsuit. Her arms behind her
back were keeping her upright, exposing her breasts.
Douglas Fairbanks was looking towards her apprecia-
tively. The photo said no more than that a famous man
looked at her, as if she were a mirror in which to check
he still had it.

To think, she said, when we were looking at the
photo, you wasn't born then. To think she could have
had . . . anyone, but now she hadn't got anything
except the photos (almost certainly burned in the flats'
furnace). It was one of the photos my mother pulled
out first when we sat down to review her past. All she
had now, penniless and homeless, was for me to marry
well somehow. Life lifted by my excellent wedding,
she as a much loved mother-in-law. Into literary life?
I don't think that was what she had in mind. It was
respectability, swagged curtains and Martinis. But all
she had was her frizzy-haired daughter with her nose
stuck in a book. It was never going to happen. She
must have known that. In the photo at her wedding my
mother was as I had never seen her, incredibly beautiful. Getting married, to a handsome young man in the
schmatter trade. But under the beauty, her eyes shone
steely. She was on her way. It was uncanny. The beauty
and the cold eyes.

This was her last chance, handing me over to a
slightly famous writer. There were possibilities, but also
the opportunity to get me off her hands. She wrote once
or twice later to say that she was going out with a very
nice Italian in the restaurant business. The picture told
of a tall, dark man in his thirties, smiling at the camera
with my mother behind it. In another letter she asked if

I'd had any Valentine cards. She'd had ten. No, I said. I hadn't had any. 'No? Well. The way you look, like a dirty beatnik.'

I don't think she thought it likely there was much room in the house, or the day, for behaving like a lady. Doris was what I'd expected of an independent woman of forty-four, a writer, a person with their own house and a son at boarding school. I don't know why I expected anything of her, I hadn't read *The Golden Notebook*, or any of the other books about women who actually lived lives. I sensed her confidence and sophistication. She exuded calm as we sipped the soup, though it turned out she felt nothing of the sort, as why should she, opening the door to an unmanageable waif and her mad mother who was much more in need of mothering. I keep finding myself on Doris's side of the door, holding Grey Kitten, my hand rising, touching the lock, but not yet turning it to let the visitors (only one of whom was just a visitor) in. I must have caught something of her panic at what she had done. For me, turning up at a stranger's house where I was to live for some time had been a pretty regular event.

When I was about the same age as Doris was then, with my own flat and daughter and an ex-husband who was my best friend, I had a long hard think about Doris then and what she had done. Her offer was immensely generous. If she had met me a few times, if we'd had coffee somewhere in Brighton, had me to stay for a few days, that would have made sense, but it would have raised expectations that might have been dashed. This was a rush into kindness. Perhaps all acts of generosity are that. Momentary acts. But where was the safety net for either of us?

I was at least as selfish as Doris. At forty-four I wanted my writer's time, alone time, and thought my life was quite full enough, although I was never very sociable. I couldn't think Doris had really thought it through, or if she had, she must have supposed that her command of human psychology was great enough to overcome any obstacles. Great arrogance, then, or in the mood for taking a chance. Or something else. Or nothing. I didn't think about her taking on a needy adolescent as an act of reparation for leaving her two children. Taking the child with no siblings. I can't say for sure, but I imagine that taking me in was much more painful for the children left behind. Why not one of them, both of them? Maybe they didn't want to come. If it was making reparation, it was a reparation of her own choosing: bright, with a capacity to learn, sassy, nobody's fool. She got that, but perhaps, like one of her characters, she supposed she could handle me. It's true that she thought I would be going away to boarding school, like Peter. So there would only be the holidays, during which, anyway, she gave up on work to accommodate Peter's presence. I think she really felt that she could cope with anything, anyone *difficult* because she wrote about such people every day, and since most of those characters were her, she would know how to manage it, and had already worked out how the relationship with me would be controlled and contained. I really don't know what she had in mind to make it work except she was still in her phase of believing that everything under the sun could be dealt with if one only understood the psychology of it. Listening, interpreting. I had, and I think she had, a sense that she knew it all. She had been pals with R. D. Laing and lived some crazed years with Clancy Sigal. She had read a bunch of Pelican books on the sociology and psychology of behaviour. We all did then, they sat on bookshop shelves like a university course: Laing, David Stafford-Clark, Erving Goffman, Vance Packard, Michael Argyle, C. J. Adcock, Viktor Frankl. And more and more. They were all over the house, on tables, on the floor. She bought them, I bought them, Peter and his friends bought them. Somehow they were cheap enough for the smallest allowance. All these were read and taken in. How could you not cope with a difficult adolescent with all that under your belt?

The answer to that was: by never having one actually there all the time, who confronted you all the time, day after day, feeling she was about to be abandoned at any moment. The worst thing in the world; but it had to be tested. Even details. What would happen if I didn't do the washing-up, what if I wore my black-and-white make-up like war paint, obscuring my face, what if I wore skirts that were the shortest I could find and then hemmed them shorter? What did I have to do, or not do, before I was sent off to . . . the wilderness? Or was I just doing what all but the most placid of children did within families checking the boundaries? Doris thought me older, perfectly able to cope with the world. I was one of those girls, more in control of myself, more a woman. I'd lived through this and that and here I was being given the opportunity to . . . what? She was always using the word 'needy', but as a criticism. I was about the neediest person in the world. She may not have known about real psychology, but needy is its Mont Blanc. It must have been awful. As I was reading pretty much the same books, Doris thought I should have learned from them how to behave. It never occurred to her that she hadn't had any hands-on practice with real-life difficult kids, or that giving them diaphragms and no stated boundaries just upped the ante. She spoke about sex to me as if I were a grown-up friend of hers, as if an experiment of equality with other people was the answer. 'They' just aren't being listened to, the reasons why 'they' split, why she'd stopped seeing A or B, what was the attraction of C with whom she was just off for a weekend, why he would do for a while after they returned. She spoke to me as near as possible as if I was her best friend. I don't think Doris knew at all what was to be done with a sulky adolescent. I understand how difficult it is, I don't think I would be able to do it, and at that point, I would have tried to find another way to help, or dropped the whole thing, just like many people would. But Doris was sure that she could.

When Peter came home for the holidays, his friends came round; he was then an alpha male, tallish, good-looking, with a mother who had interesting people round at her house in London. We hung out upstairs, listening to music, talking about our worries, and during supper in the kitchen some of us would continue to talk about them with Doris there. She enjoyed this role, as we see in *The Sweetest Dream*. The surrogate mother. The adult who understood. There were also too many interesting adolescents (and stray cats, and crazy old women from the North Wing, St Pancras knocking on the door and being given cups of tea until the police came) around for us to notice if Peter in particular was OK. He had learned from a young age how to act like one of the grown-ups. He talked forcefully but he didn't know that much. And Doris stopped arguments between him and others (often me). 'Oh that's enough. You're so boring. Let's get on to something else.' Soon enough Peter found himself a catchphrase: 'What you don't understand, Jen, is that we are both saying the same thing, and you are agreeing with me.' Like three-year-old Jennifer, I wasn't going to let that go by, and answered: 'We *aren't* talking about the same thing.' We were irritating teenagers, in my case, sitting around someone else's mother's table being miserable. We hated the Bomb, we hated education as it was done at school, we hated apartheid. We hated families. Doris made quantities of food and enjoyed her role as a liberal adult. Then Peter and everyone else would go back to boarding school or their homes, and I remained in Charrington Street. Peter didn't obviously 'present', as they say, as a deeply troubled young man, until a few years later.

I was there all the time and had no real idea what to do. For all Doris's talks about sex and politics, I felt there was more to know in a different way. I was on the lookout for older men (not hard to find) to teach me about adult sex, and what they knew about the world. Doris – who never explained why, despite providing me with a diaphragm, I wasn't supposed to bring men home to have sex with in my bedroom – was not a very reliable source of wisdom. I was moody, which was and always had been my character, as I thought, rather than badly behaved. I couldn't believe that Doris, who seemed to have had similar moods, wouldn't understand. But I'm often told by the few people still around from that time that I was terribly 'difficult'. Some of them also tell me I have got some of the details here wrong, but they are my details, my experience, and I've learned to trust my memory rather than theirs. I've tried very hard to think about what I actually did wrong: smoking, having sex, using dope, not working hard enough, staying out late at night. But I don't know anyone who hasn't had some or all of that from their teenagers. The question remained, the one that had been there since I first arrived: if Doris didn't like me, what was she going to do with me? And the answer was that I'd get thrown out when I was more than Doris could stand. Doris wanted a young person she could deal with and make better with bowls of soup, and for it to be understood that I'd been taken under the wing of an incredibly insightful woman. But I wasn't Laing's sort of patient. I didn't hallucinate, I just threw myself against the walls and discovered that they weren't rubber, but shattered fairly easily. I was doing sex, staying out late, spending too much money on things that weren't sensible, being moody and silent at supper parties. I argued with Peter when he was there. I don't think it was very much more than that, this shocking behaviour. And all of it could have been fixed by telling me not to.

At any rate, she raced to get me to see a psychologist at the Tavistock Clinic and got one for Peter, too. It seems they didn't help much with my awfulness and what was to come from Peter. She took us away from the Tavistock when she went to see Peter's therapist and found he wanted to look into Peter's childhood parenting. Joan Rodker had letters from Doris around then, which, at Doris's request, she embargoed until after my death. Almost tragically, this very talented but blocked painter couldn't get rid of the pain she felt at having been ostracised by Doris after she told Doris that she thought Peter was a catastrophe that wouldn't have happened had she got him proper treatment. Even near the very end of her life, in her nineties, Joan wept about Peter. She offered to unembargo Doris's letters for me, so that I could read them. But I knew pretty much what would be in them, and how little I would benefit from it. Joan agreed and said mostly they were complaints about my behaviour, the men, not working hard enough for my A-levels and most of all my ingratitude.

There were three major external influences in Doris's life. The first, communism, lasted until 1956, when like many people, she left the Party. That period is laid out in great detail in *The Golden Notebook* (Joan is there, answering the phone, sitting on the bottom stair by the kitchen, both in real life and in the novel): a powerful thing about Doris's earlier novels, including *The Golden Notebook* and *The Four-Gated City*, is that they present a period and a certain kind of thinking of the time accurately; not so much the later books, such as *The Good Terrorist*, which also presents people she knew, but shockingly and, I think, faithlessly disguised by using them to tell a story that she knew very little about. The second, psychology, was waning by the time I arrived, and Doris had discovered Sufism. She had been looking around the specialist occult bookshops like Watkins, and going to meetings of various groups that claimed they had the real truth about our planet. She did some hatha yoga and stood on her head every day, and read and spoke to fellow browsers in the bookshops. Finally she came up with a group called Subud; a 'real' teacher was about to arrive in England and set up teaching groups from the shards left behind in Paris and London after Gurdjieff died. This one coming – Idries Shah, as it turned out – was the real thing. A world teacher, Doris told me excitedly. I asked how she would know, but she was intuitively sure that the people at Subud had their fingers on the pulse. Still, how would she know he really was 'the' teacher, and not just another guru, of whom there were already some, and who would become a raga-storm as the 1960s moved towards their end?

That was the point, Doris said, one *would* know if one allowed oneself to be insightful and not emotional. The mind had to be made ready, sensitive enough with preparation.

Mescaline was legal at the time, and the manufacturers in Switzerland were giving it away to 'artists and writers'. I recall a long day sitting in my room listening to screams and dramatic laughter down below as two friends in the occult business took her through 'rebirthing'. It was as scary for me as it was for Doris, I think. I wasn't sure she wasn't dead or mad for evermore until the next day. In the meantime, I went to school and didn't do enough work for my A-levels, spent most of my school day in the café in the park opposite and met lovers at lunchtime, while Doris read and listened to teaching stories and did whatever exercises they did to open up their hearts/minds to the truth. In the evenings she would tell me the latest news from the metaphysical world.

Sufism lasted, as far as I can tell, for the rest of Doris's conscious life. In later years she never spoke to me about 'the Work', as it was called. I wasn't sure whether this was from disappointment about the teaching or from her understanding that I was a failure and therefore to be kept in the dark. She told me when Shah died of heart failure in 1996, but only for my information. No questions allowed. No weeping, no distress. After all, we were all here on borrowed time, waiting for the penny to drop. Shah set up groups and organisations, and Roger, our small daughter and I often spent a Saturday or Sunday first in his house in a leafy village not too far from London and then at Langton House near Tunbridge Wells, another suburb of perfect respectability. The house was, I suppose, formerly the old landowner's house, large and walled, with outbuildings and a huge garden. Things were various. People in groups went at weekends to manicure the gardens and on Saturday night to have a group meal and listen to Shah's table talk, which was, if you listened properly, Doris said, his real teaching. There were public lectures, generally on historical or philosophical topics. The lecturers were academics or highly regarded journalists and writers, who, as far as I know, had nothing to do with the Sufis, or even knew that they were speaking under their aegis, but were paid to lecture by the Institute for Cultural Research, set up by Shah. Sometimes I thought that there were secret Sufis, dotted around the place keeping the planet from exploding. I remember a lecture about Vico, a lecture by Richard Gregory on the physiology of perception, for all the world as if a Pelican book had come to life, and a rather baffled aged British traveller to Eastern Parts, who talked with all the ease of his upbringing of 'fuzzywuzzies' while I squeezed someone's hand in order to contain my embarrassment. A mixed bunch, but not at all uninteresting and nothing to do with the occult. There were what seemed to be Women's Institute days, when people brought and sold cakes and biscuits, and tea was available from an urn.

We were marshalled along by Doris, sometimes instructed to take one of her irritating adoratas from California or thereabouts in our car. They spoke of Doris as if she were a source of wisdom, and her every move significant and the car journeys felt very long. But it all seemed harmless, and as I said interesting in its spotty way. Part of the teaching is that the teaching is scattered among the quotidian tasks of life. That didn't seem too terrible an idea. My daughter enjoyed the trips to Langton, and made a firm weekly friend of a boy about the same age. They were often asked to pick out the winner of the raffle on stage. Once or twice there were full-blown parties, the first a 'three-day party' inside the grounds of the house, which I remember as hypnotic fun: at three a.m. with everything slow and sleepy, Ward Swingle, who started the a cappella group, sat down at the piano in the food tent and began to play and sing 'September Song'. That *was* something.

For all I could see, apart from Doris going off to weekly 'meetings', weekends gardening and having the weekend meal, and meditating every Thursday for an hour, when I sometimes joined her in front of a mandala, it was a reasonable way to fill up a life without getting in the way of work (it was a while before the Sufi beliefs fully showed up in Doris's books as 'inner space fiction'). 'It's not meditating,' she would say firmly as we began to breathe deeply and evenly. 'We are still in nursery school. This is just learning to concentrate.' This also made sense to me. We were doing elementary mindfulness as we would think of it now: counting breaths as we looked at the mandala and watching out for thoughts which we noticed and let pass like clouds, not allowing ourselves to dwell on them. I still do it (minus the mandala) under its umbrella as mindfulness. It's handy, helps with pain and sometimes depression. At least while you're doing it. As to the groups that Shah told Doris I wasn't stable enough to attend, Doris never mentioned what went on in them, though she often gave out the news Shah dropped during his Saturday evening after-dinner table talk, in which there was more apparently than met the eye. Like our being overrun by the Russians and then the Chinese. Bombs would fall, civilisation would end. Quite like most TV series now, it was all quietly but firmly apocalyptic.

One hilarious day, Doris turned up with a sagging plastic bag of silver ingots. About eight of them, which she handed to me. She had also given Peter a bagful. 'These are for when it gets really bad. People will always want silver and you can exchange it for food.' I was stunned: people would exchange food for lumps of silver? I said that someone would need them more and I would exchange my teaching experience for a bowl of porridge and I didn't want them. She insisted, so that my daughter and I would survive. (She must have cared for me in some way.) I used two or three as paperweights and doorstops, and within barely a month or so, the bottom fell out of silver.

Doris told me these things because she didn't have anyone else nearby who wouldn't laugh and she wasn't supposed to discuss the meetings with others in the group. Sometime earlier she said I shouldn't tell a mutual friend of ours about the forthcoming end of the world, because it would be hard for a 'young woman with a baby to take it'. Although ten years younger, I evidently could because I didn't have a baby. I suppose she was right. I hadn't had a child then. I listened and then waited for the world to end. Doris taking Russian A-level arose from this, so she could 'read the signposts'. I declined to join her, but Peter was brought in on it. At the end of the course Doris got an A and Peter failed. Another needless cruelty. From then on Peter went deeper into fantasy, telling Doris's admirers that he was a physicist or CEO of some groundbreaking company. He started using 'we' about Doris's books and her agents and publishers. Most of her friends were now from her Russian course. When that finished, most of them stopped being visitors.

When I thought I'd better get off the drugs I was taking, Doris (who regarded me as Lazarus having risen from the dead at this point) offered me the small basement flat in her house. I asked about joining one of Shah's groups. The idea of being cut loose from all my society, plus dumping mind-calming drugs, scared me. A nice study group seemed just the thing. In the druggy world, I was part of something, really for the first time. I discovered I could inject speed and sit in a room with other people and feel I belonged. Well . . . That was when the message came back from Shah via Doris that I was not 'psychologically stable enough' to belong to a group. So – oh Jesus – I had to prove my stability. This was the 'learning to be a secretary and get a job' period. I couldn't think of anything more stable to do. I wasn't much good. Deference didn't work for me, nor did making cups of tea, or having to pretend that I had a full day's work, when actually it could all be done in two hours and the rest of the day had to be spent pretending to be busy. Only a year or so later, tired of waiting for approbation, I thought, like many others in the 1970s, that teaching 'hopeless' kids in a 'hopeless' school was about the most useful thing I could do. I went to a teacher training college (no A-levels, or degree, so I had to get a teaching certificate) and landed in a comprehensive school in Hackney full of wild and angry young women. These days it's a monument to good working practices, but then, when Hackney wasn't the Hackney anyone under my age could imagine, it was more a matter of social work, ducking chairs and getting classes of thirty calm enough to listen to what sometimes appealed to them. Mostly information about their bodies and sex.

After Shah died, it wasn't clear whether the Work was continuing or not. I'm fairly sure I'd let her down by not devoting myself to getting right for the Work. I'd given up and thought there wasn't anything I could do where being a nut job didn't mosey along beside me whatever I did. Nor did I think I very much wanted to be part of 'all that'. Online they say that Shah had said that all the teaching was in his books. So I suppose the groups went on as I've described, or they collapsed. Perhaps a little of both. Perhaps that was what Doris meant when she said to a friend, who passed it on, that as far as she was concerned, taking drugs and living my own life, I was already dead. Or she meant exactly what she said. There really wasn't much in Shah's teaching to complain about. It required some work, reading, thinking, some entertaining stories, no mention of God or Allah to frighten modern Westerners away, while providing some pleasant public functions. There was an embargo on being social with one another outside of the Work, but most of Doris's friends were now involved in the Work – partly because those who sniffed at Shah as a charlatan (there were plenty about) were ousted from Doris's address book. 'Well, he/she had their chance,' Doris would shrug. It felt pitiless. From time to time she would say to me, crossly, that they weren't there to have fun together but to learn.

There was really only one thing that made me firmly keep away from 'the Work'. When Peter was about thirty, so in the mid-1970s, I said to Doris that Peter was in a terrible state, overweight, taking no exercise, speaking nonsense, and shouldn't she try and get him to see someone. She said that *they* were all charlatans, and in any case, there was nothing wrong with Peter psychologically; and then she said that Shah had specifically told her that she should leave Peter to stay home and do nothing because when he became forty he would come right. He'd seen it happen before. This, I think, remained Doris's justification for keeping Peter in their small flat and then buying him a flat next to her larger new house. A door was knocked through between Doris's kitchen and the hallway outside Peter's bedroom, so he didn't have far to walk for breakfast. Peter's fortieth birthday came and went. He became alarmingly anti-social, walked around without trousers or pants, shat where he stood or sat, abused women and generally anyone standing in his eyeline, and essentially turned into the monstrous baby that someone (he or Doris) wanted him to be. Who to blame for that? Doris and Shah; even if I have no right to be angry, even if it was my fault for ousting him from the nest, or in this case keeping him in the nest – for not even trying. And of course, it's not my business, as I was told by Doris, who was telling everyone that it was. Going to visit her, even after she had had the stroke that left her smiley and virtually wordless, the old nameless fury bubbled up as my feet hit the pavement, walking towards their house or the hospital, and came to a peak as I rang the doorbell, latterly bringing cakes, as all her visitors did. Peter by then was diabetic and had a district nurse come in to give him insulin injections, but before her stroke, Doris was feeding him exactly what diabetics are supposed not to eat, chocolates, sticky puddings, potatoes, squash, heavy stews, cake, though later she kept the cake for herself, pulling it to her in case anyone else thought they were getting any. Once Doris had her stroke and they both had full-time carers in, they were more careful with his diet.

Shah was charismatic, attractive, charming and some-times stern. One long weekend, before he died, I found myself surrounded by shocked people who were off to spend three days walking with their light bags towards the buried sewer pipe where Shah and a Welsh university had asked volunteers to spend three (I think) days, in order to test humidity and CO_2 levels, while also being a demonstration of how small isolated groups work. When Roger said he couldn't go I took his place. (This was the occasion when Shah asked me if I thought he was a male chauvinist pig for offering to carry my bag. That was the full extent of my conversations with Shah.) The stay in the sewer pipe was interesting mainly for the almost clockwork way in which everyone behaved accord-ing to the textbooks: leadership locking of horns from alpha males, women presiding over making the place *nice* and getting the 'food' ready (pot noodles mostly). It was another by-law of the Work that it wasn't to be judged by its followers, but it did for me. On the last day, when suggestions for improvements were being listed, one of the women suggested it would be a good idea if women wore pink and men wore blue. 'So we can tell them apart,' I muttered, having no inkling of the coming gender-queer furore, and then bit my tongue. One thing you don't do in small secluded groups is show dismay. It was to circumvent any aggression, she said. I certainly needed colour coding, my aggression levels were going through the steel roof. I wrote her suggestion down in the diary I'd agreed to keep and mentally disappeared into a novel. Where was the wisdom in these people who had been going to groups and meditating for decades before

Shah arrived? If you can't tell anything about a mystical group by its adherents, how else are you to judge it? Of course there were the silent Sufis, living in the world (not of it), making sure that things didn't get out of hand, which was why, Doris said, the Cold War had not erupted into a killing fest. Also, the crumbs under my bed keep the elephants away.

What I started disliking more and more about the Sufis was that sense of belonging to an elite, of a small group of people – most of them privately educated and wealthy – who thought they had access to a secret that others didn't, and who were smiling patronisingly as one smiles at a child. Rather like the Sufi who, on hearing of Doris's death just weeks after Peter's, told me that at last they were together for ever. That was a shocker. Peter was never to get away from his mother, not even in eternity. I disliked this petty confidence so much that I had already given strict instructions to people around me that Doris was not to be allowed anywhere near my deathbed, even if it meant barricading the doors. As it turned out, I needn't have worried. Here I am, on my death sofa, with Doris gone before, and in Cambridge, where any other deathbed-lovers from my time with the Sufis would have a slightly more difficult job getting to me.

———————

I'm not as fond of David Bowie as most people seem to be. I'm certainly not dancing a reel in the streets. Some good songs, an enviable capacity to shapeshift, but not so much charm, or humility, as some who nevertheless die young, younger, with children and grandchildren to leave. But that more than anything made me tear up during the tribute programmes. What distressed him most about dying, said this icon of narcissism once, was the thought of missing watching his daughter grow up: 'It just doubles me up in a kind of grief.' That's certainly the key that gets the endocrine glands flowing down my cheeks. That's the unbearable loss. Everything else can be made sense of. The loss of the future children and grandchildren is unbearable, although quite in order, quite in the way of things. It's as simple as pushing a button, and I'm lost in no man's land. The insoluble grief. Not that there's anything to be done about any of it.

Doris died, at home. She caught an infection, and was left unmedicated as she had wished. We got her a hospital bed and the local palliative care team looked after her. She became increasingly comatose until she stopped breathing one morning and was pronounced dead. It was that afternoon that one of the Sufis phoned to assure me that Peter and Doris would always be together. I wasn't in my most graceful frame of mind. 'Dear Christ, I hope not!' I had a picture of Doris gunning it up towards Peter, and each failing ever to get away from the other. Like the Pleiades. Always away from and towards their doom, shrieking, 'Will you never leave me alone?', while they fruitlessly fled for the hills, hiding behind a passing cloud (those beautiful cigarette packets in a lovely shade of pink and gentle clouds of smoke) and running for them there hills, saying: 'Leave me be. Even here? What have I done?' While a voice boomed: 'You didn't make enough effort; no, scratch that, you'll never get away, you didn't fight for your freedom when you had it.' Oh lord, what a terrible vision. Out and then in. Each dying then recovering.

While they were both still in hospital, my daughter Chloe and I would meet waiting for the elevator between their separate floors, have a quick grim consultation with each other about the two days of life Peter was expected to have left. 'Well, what happens happens,' Doris said when we told her, a phrase we would never have imagined her using. We were taken aback a moment, and then went our trusted ways up and down the lifts, to arrange a 'final' goodbye. 'I've never done this before,' I said nervously, to Chloe. A small bark of humanity passed between us. But by the time the hoist for Peter's eating arrangements was sorted out, the crisis was over and Peter was pronounced living for a day or two more. We, Doris's staples – Roger, Chloe, Christopher (another waif who turned up for hot meals and rescue) and I – took it in turns to wait outside the ICU, to be called, at that point we didn't know if we were doing it for Doris or Peter, or simply to assuage guilty feelings. What was his quality of life? The big question from the doctor who made the big decisions. None of us could find a good or even reasonable answer, just looked at each other (having varying qualities of our own lives), but the big doc perhaps interpreted our willingness to be there as quality in his life and ticked the box marked 'good enough'. So on it went until first Peter, then Doris decided on the quality of their lives and proceeded to get on with them at home. My guess is that Peter decided he'd won by dying first, and Doris that she'd be damned if he was going to get away from her that easily. A gracefully executed ending, even leaving time for Doris's daughter to arrive for the eulogy.

But back to me (it's not all about me, I know, but some of it is). I spent a week or so as a patient before and after Christmas at Addenbrooke's. One day I had a fever and was speaking in tongues, and Chloe and the Poet thought I was dying, although, as I pointed out, just to announce that one is a cucumber doesn't count as consent to termination. But I didn't die because they got the drip feed under my skin and poured their potion of antibiotics in fast enough. I was a bit mad for a day or two. 'A bit?' muttered the Poet. 'A *bit* mad!' my sterner daughter exploded. Well more than a bit. I had weird dreams which didn't go away even when they woke me up. I was in some North African war, trying to save my daughter from being abducted and no one was going to stop me. Or I was trying to get the Poet out of prison for writing unnecessary poetry. Then I'd phone him at around three in the morning to see if they were lying to me. It took about three days to get out of that dream. The Poet put up with it as kindly as anyone woken at three in the morning would.

So I was not compos mentis and had no idea where 'I' was. Usually it was prison. Daytimes I was generally OK, though a bit knackered with all my night-time battles. Woke up, had pills, had Weetabix and something like a shower. Then in a clean nightie I was ready to face the day. Not that most people thought that banging away at my computer was much in the way of work, and, let's face it, I wasn't knitting socks for our boys at the front. Wherever that was. The lady chaplain came round, but I said she'd do better praying for God himself; he had after all, caused all the trouble. One crap in the world and it was time to clear up the fucking mess he'd made of it. We were at least owed an apology.

Mostly I wrote sitting up in bed, a condition I prefer. Beds were made for everyday living. The nurses were very kind and chucked me under the chin as if I were six. I thought I might stay there, but more and more people came to die – the hospice was full – and anyway apart from the clean sheets, home suited my needs. After seven days I said I was going home.

'Why?'

'Because apart from lung cancer and fibrosis I now have a hospital-borne infection which no one knows how to cure. I am going home.' I have enough knowledge of how institutions work to know that I had just to sound as if I knew what they did and did not have a right to do, and they were not doing it to me.

'We won't let you go.'

'You can't stop me.'

'Yes, we can.'

Without going into the ins and outs of the law on sectioning, I related, quietly and not at all as if I were about to kill someone, the necessary conditions for sectioning people. No danger to herself or others, to qualified doctors, etc., to make me sound like trouble. She backed away and, behold, there was another route to keeping everyone happy. Well, if not happy, at least without dogfood on anyone's snout. A line was inserted from my upper arm to my heart, into which large daily doses of antibiotic were to be injected while I sat in the kitchen or my bed. So I am home and they have got rid of a potentially annoying patient. Always a simple answer to a dangerous argument, which could have left everyone waiting to fight the good fight.

If only I'd known this when I was at war with the management (aka nurses) all those years ago in the Maudsley. Now, aged 68, I find myself back in the same old discourse, them gently enticing or threatening, or us, like startled chimps, pushed into a cave with a banana as an edible treat. Once we had a handle on the thing it was too late. Now, decades on, I had to learn the old tricks again. Placate but make it clear you know how the rules are enforced and that you know how to enforce them, but you have to remain calm. The worst thing is to put them in a defensive position, because then there is nowhere to go and nothing for them to do but rattle their keys like sabres.

I was back home with my 'package of care' and the kind of satisfaction someone feels who has found the crack in the wall where the tiny key fits and lets us out. There were no battles to be won or lost, just medications and pulses. Perhaps not as effective as pills in a hospital, but not tensed or straining against idiot rules designed to make the nursing staff not responsible for anything. I am willing to do anything to keep away from their keys which bring with them the pills that space out time like a clock. I eat Weetabix, have sitting-down showers, let them thread plastic lines to my heart to guggle down huge quantities of antibiotics, all in the name of keeping out of their clutches. 'Disinhibited', the Poet calls it. But just get an inch inside my defences and they'll see what granite I'm made of.

In the meantime, I'm warm, not to say cosy, and my time, such as it is, is my own. But warm and comfortable seems good, at least not horrified with constant thoughts of death. I do think constantly of death, my death, the only one I'll have. They are closing the ring of wagons as I watch and feel for symptoms. But there are too many to be worried. A pain in my side, high/low blood pressure, tiredness, anything happening in my body and mind could be the cancer, or the fibrosis, or the pneumonia or the fear of some other symptom hiding in the woods pretending to be a tree. So I think I'd better not be afraid, I'll always be afraid.

But I am scared of dissolution, of casting my particles to the wind, of having nothing to cast my particles to the wind with, of knowing nothing when knowing everything has been the taste every day, little by little, by knowing what little meant compared to a lot, compared to something or nothing. People have always worried me with questions, questions have always worried me with having no answers. That's what I mean. I don't know enough, or know nothing. And then I get to the nub of it. What should I know about? When great minds have gone to dust, what could it possibly matter what I know or don't know? What arrogance to imagine that my minute fossils of knowledge are of any importance. Then again who is going to win the Third World War? How will my grandchildren manage in a world that is daily dispersing, without a grandmother who has already dispersed? Or most simply, I'm curious. What will I not know when I'm not a knowing machine? There are too many questions for an ordinary curious mind. How can nothing be nothing? Help me out here, philosophers, there isn't much time. Or is it really just a dance, a quadrille made from the soup of Alice's tears. Alice doesn't have tears. Well, that's what you know. I've done a backstroke in those tears. Want a race?

I'm very feeble but no longer going to die of pneumonia, apparently. So here I am, thinking and taking pills, wondering whether the fibrosis will kill me first or the tumour. The feeling that my death was waiting on the doorstep with the milk bottles has lessened. It was Christmas, and probably my last, and I've been practising my grand grumpitude to ensure that my grandchildren think 'bah' as effectively as their irascible Granjen. At this rate I'll be dying like a dearest grandmama would with a grin from here to here. Swinging from the whirling light that Hitchcock made everyone scream about.

I've been given one last chance. A trial pill (probably filled with sugar) I'm to take every day, no fat or anything nice in my diet. The last lot I stopped because they made me sick and miserable, and generally gave me very little quality of life. Qualia: do you love it or hate it? These new ones have bad side-effects after which there is 'nothing we can do for you', said the nice doctor at Papworth. The paper you get with the pills said an agonising pain in the upper abdomen was possible. I was having goose for Christmas, so I'd decided not to take them until after Boxing Day. And then I got sick. About half a dozen people have been diagnosed or died of cancer the last few weeks, so cancer has a bit of a domestic ring about it. (No, Clive James is still with us.)

Incidentally, anyone wanting to send me a late Christmas sorry-you're-dying prezzie, I want a silk or organic cashmere something, so I can waft my way through the box sets and die happy at having seen the last episode of *The Bridge 3* in cosy things that I can stroke – there is the Poet but it's not the same as a dead goat. Top of my list (after the sumptuous silk) is that our neighbours not start building work till I'm gone. Or at least stop them playing Radio 1.

I don't think I want a funeral. Very last year. But it can take up some usefully distracting argumentation. Always fancied 'Smoke Gets in Your Eyes' and for the Poet to sing a properly political song – maybe, like at my old friend Joan's funeral, 'The Ballad of Joe Hill', and that Tallahassee song so perhaps I'll know what she threw over the bloody bridge. And finally 'Me and Bobbie McGee'. Also, come to think of it, the Grosse Fuge. OK, that's it for now.

For several days now I've been feeling as if I'm on a holiday, a short one coming to its end. Not an especially good one. Not sorry to be leaving, not sorry to have been here. No particular feeling one way or another. Not living in my place. Not familiar enough. As one might sit on the edge of a chair that is waiting for another occupant to take it over. It's the strangest of strange feelings. Best travelling clothes, a ticking of a clock that will go on ticking after you leave and after the next occupant too. An especially powerful image that. The clock that clicks as generation after generation passes by. And all along a narcissistic metric that keeps the haphazardest of lives seeming to be afloat on an even keel. It is, of course, the ticking, tocking of this everlasting, or outlasting, clock that keeps everything seeming so orderly, that is, you realise, keeping the time.

About time too, someone says in the distance, and you realise that it is about time. Catch a handful of salted peanuts, then pick up your cheap suitcase for the forward journey. There must have been hope at the start, thoughts of something, exciting or eventful, and now it's time to be going home. Back to the real familiarity that the holiday was taken from. The real break in the everyday, every – what would you call it? So I'm sitting here on the moquette, ankles close together to take the journey home. An adventure the other way.

Well, that is my sense of death and the station platform waiting for the train and its slow delay. It doesn't matter a jot now, in my actual place. But the overwhelming importance of loss and necessity in the background that keeps what ought to keep always ticking, and also always steady. A steadiness keeping the one thing and the other apart.

You've done it now. Vanilla on your clean white gloves and shoes. Each way, for some reason no one will explain, the whiteness of gloves and shoes – the shoes painted with a chalky white substance that had to be waited for to dry. One scuff and the story's told, the mystery is out. But not to me. Why, when it is so unimportant, is the whiteness of the shoes essential? Who could possibly keep these gloves and shoes white, at the dirtiest part of the journey? Why should it matter? Do you want them (who?) to think you have magical properties that keep pure the extremes of the body most likely to pick up dirt from floor and ticket booths? What could it possibly pain anyone to see a scuff mark on the inside of the top left of a shoe front? What a lovely child. So clean, so nicely kept. What a paragon of a mother that formulaic child must have. How carefully I folded the whites of my clothing when I crossed the road and slipped through the wire fence to the bomb site. Put my carefully folded clothes on the flattest, cleanest stone I could find, so that I could run around, play houses, my knickers' elastic broken and pulled so I could put some in my mouth and chew elastically on it. Then return home after my mysterious play at housework, as clean as any school day, as any child could achieve. A ritual. Building the walls. Three bricks high, openings for doors and windows. Or perhaps I am lying against myself, only wishing to wrinkle and make dirty the dirtiness of my floppy knickers. (That part was true, I did nibble on my dirty knicker elastic, forever a mystery to my mother. How could a child arrive from a day at school with grubby, broken knicker elastic?) She had no nose for the most pointless of activities. For the delicacies of all delicacies, broken knicker elastic. Perhaps no one did. Or no one apart from me. 'Eugh, she's eating broken knicker elastic. That's well dirty.' I couldn't know. It never occurred to me to find out.

With carefully wiped hands I returned to my pile of clothing, put the clothes on in the correct order, as exact as if we were a family with varying places on the OCD chart (we were, of course). My mother looking over every part of me to find the source of the problem. This way, that, don't leave anything out. Sniffing through my well-worn clothes that would prove definitively I was one of those dirty children she would not have her child playing with.

'Why can't I play with them?'

'Because they're dirty.'

But they were no more dirty than I was.

They touched things. I imagined some things I could touch, but couldn't come up with anything I hadn't touched already. Was there a sneaking place? A hidden place that no one knew about but everyone touched that made them 'dirty'? I wished I could find the dirty place, so hidden that no one would find it. That only I knew about. And only I thought of to play with. But nothing was so secret, so hidden that one couldn't see it. Where was it? What did it do? But my mother's investigations were so carefully done nothing could have been missed. Oh, you pretty things. Go to another place to find what you are looking for. I was my mother's prettiest thing, but was only told to leave the room occasionally, and then it was so she could swear and curse the day she and I had been born. So the secret, if not the activity, was and remained a mystery to me for a long time.

Illness, as normal people understand it, was virtually prohibited in my flat of two rooms. You got shouted at if you had a temperature. No more or less shouted at than any other affair that meant difficulty for her. When I was eleven she arrived at the boarding school where the combined efforts of the local education authority and social services had sent me. She had a white paper bag, and inside, spoken of in undertones, was a pink plastic box. She'd been to the doctor, she said, and he said it was all right to start now. You can shave yourself, maybe twice a month, your lower legs. Just like an ordinary shaver, but smaller. It seemed that I was medically approved to do my legs and under my arms. But I wasn't ill. It wasn't a treatment. And this is how life went on. A year or so later I had my first period, known as being 'unwell', where mostly you sat on a sofa and took two aspirin every four hours. She would have to slap my face when it first started. The strangest of all the medications. But when it actually happened it seemed as if she needed to be slapped in the face, so appalled and panicked was she. All that, I learned very much later, was part of Jewish tradition. Face-slapping. And keeping 'clean', making evil take its place at the back of the schul. Jewish stuff, women's stuff. Who knew, who cared? What would happen to me if a curl of hair was found in the bathroom? This was all folkloric stuff, but very hard to separate from the mad rituals of my mother, who, as far as I know, carried on her own mad fancies with little regard for the cleansing ritual that tried to make clean what the Lord made dirty every month, to say nothing of the Lord and his tabernacles, whatever *they* turned out to be.

It was my mother's middle-aged panic acting out in me. I lay on the sofa with an upturned hand over my forehead as I'm sure they were depicted in *Little Women*, while Marmee took hot, freshly baked rolls to poor families in a basket under a gingham cloth. It was entirely weird and disturbing to try putting these certainties also under the cloth with the white rolls. Unwell, after all, is not ill, nor, as far as I know, did red gingham do much for stomach cramps. The mishmash suddenly made the only sense, mishmash whirled around and pulled together in a kind of Disney dance, which hasn't been made, but should have been because it's a much better story than *Beauty and the Beast*.

AFTERWORD

The Poet

When you live in a house with somebody else, they're always there, even when they're not physically present, in ways that can be distracting, reassuring, sociable, comforting or completely annoying. Today, almost five months after Jenny's death, something of this is still true, though in a much more sorrowful way. I've grown accustomed to her absence, but the house is full of reminders, things that can jolt me into tears or flood me with delight at unexpected (and sometimes unsuitable) moments. When Jenny was alive, we used to talk all the time, about everything, inexhaustibly. Looking back, I think of that as the texture and fabric of our lives together, that and writing. And talking about writing. Or not talking about it, as sometimes you can't, or don't want to.

The best way to illustrate that is probably by using Jenny's own words which, funny and self-deprecating as they can be, are also true to the constant mystery and difficulty of love. She wrote the two short pieces of prose that follow, and published them on her blog, in 2007, just before and on her sixtieth birthday. I'd been particularly annoying for several days as her birthday approached. The house is full of books, and I'd already spent about two whole days standing in front of banks of shelves, investigating some fourteen hundred novels as part of the work of the poem I was composing for her. I was getting on Jenny's nerves and in a way quite enjoying it. Jenny wasn't enjoying it. There's nothing more unsettling than feeling someone hanging around within earshot, doing something you aren't part of. It points up the difficult gaps and differences and anxieties that always exist between lovers, and points to the leaps we try to make to get across the gaps. And if you're trying to work it's very distracting. But for a fuller explanation of what was going on, I'll let Jenny speak for herself.

The Poet has a project and it's secret. That's the thing about poets, they can have projects and spend several days wandering around the house, gazing at shelves, opening and closing books, going 'Hmmm,' 'Yes, that's good,' 'No, that won't do,' 'Well, possibly,' and when politely asked what the fuck he is doing, tell you, 'It's a project. I don't know if it's going to work yet so I can't tell you about it. I'll know by next week. I'll tell you then.' It's remarkably aggravating and full of mystery, hard thinking and purpose, all three of which are so lacking in my own prosaic doings.

When I'm thinking about writing something, I have the decency to keep him up all night talking about it, demanding his full attention at three in the morning, teasing out the maybes and possibles and then losing interest entirely. That way, he's always included in my thinking. None of this poetic withholding. He has such an aura of deep brooding about his sodding Project, whereas I plod on, page after page ('Thank God, that's 60,000 words, not so many more to go'), month after month, wailing and moaning about not being able to write, getting it wrong, taking too long, wondering what on earth I'm doing. Monday, the Poet will know what he's doing and if it's going to work; Friday, it'll be finished. And what's more it'll be a poem, which is so much more serious a thing than a novel.

And on top of that, as if being a poet and having a secret project wasn't cool and superior enough, he's downstairs baking a coffee and walnut cake for my birthday. It's insupportable.

———

All is revealed. The Poet's project worked, it turned out, but not until he'd examined over a thousand novels to find what he was looking for, while I padded (part of the time) behind him yelling, 'What the fuck are you doing?' It also turned out that it was a poem for my birthday. Ooops. It was related to the present he gave me (as if a poem wasn't enough): an etching of a rectangle divided into four on white paper in a white frame, by Linda Karshan. So beautiful and exactly what I want to look at. Also somewhat like a window on a window. The poem is below. His byzantine method of making the poem is explained in a note at the end.

Also, the cake was alarmingly delicious.

———

60 Windows

for Jenny Diski, on her sixtieth birthday

Tiny room whose window was never opened
Curtain for the window
On the cane chair under the window

Pale green even in the window
Emptying the basin out of the window
Halts by the window and gazes

Lay on the ground under the window
Kneeling up to the window
An octagonal vaulted chamber with a balconied
   window

Her bed had its back to the window
Through the curtainless window day stole in
She went to the other window

Sitting at the table near the window, working
Opened windows into the wrong world
A gale, exploding against the window

Awnings lowered outside the windows
A reproduction of a stained-glass-window angel
Whistling up at vague windows

Got up and went to the window. It was raining
   again.
Early light, coming through the uncurtained window
With its tiny windows looking on to the street

Pat wandered from the window and took up the
   George Moore novel
He came out through the French windows
She got up and stood at the window

There was moonlight in the window
There's a sharp rapping at the window
I am in the window, smoking

They had seen it happen from a window
Then went to the window that looked on the street
   below
Watching you from the apartment window

In my memory, at the window
The rain was still thudding against the window-pane
I think that I might open the window

A camera is being held to the window
Silver things in the window
From the street the windows were in darkness

His reflection could be seen in the front window
High up, from one of the small barred windows
His right arm through the open window

I put all the lamps on and opened all the windows
A huge wall broken by gaping windows loomed
   above
Sordid glare of shop windows, made beautiful by
   distance

A board nailed across a broken window
They opened all the windows
Sat and sewed by the window in the clear autumn
   afternoon

The room was almost in darkness, the windows
    quite covered
The night I stared at from my window
A castle whose windows were glittering orange squares

The windows, between lengths of white embossed
    satin
Our windows, on the second floor, overlooked the
    street
The butcher pulled down black window shades

She had been sitting in her own window
The inner courtyard on to which my window looked
    out
The middle one of the three windows was half way
    open

The sun filtered through the windows with remark-
    able subtlety
Rushed to the window, not to sail out of it
No lights behind its white painted windows

Has to look out of the window at the elements, at
    nature
Draw down the upper frame of the window
The windows were shuttered. But there was a crack.

*'60 Windows' is composed entirely of phrases that mention windows,
taken from page 60 of sixty different novels.*

The Daughter

Mum first told me about her diagnosis at her local pub in Cambridge. It was a very hot day in May and I was there with my son, Louis. The pub had a pig and a few toys for Louis to wheel about on. He was two, and wanted attention, but so did Mum, and when I had got Louis interested enough in a toy to sit with her and talk, she said without a pause or any build-up, that she had inoperable cancer. I felt dizzy, and sick, and resentful of her for telling me in such a public place with a child to look after and be okay for. Mum looked so depressed, her body shrunk to a knot of despair, not unfamiliar and really not much worse than she had seemed during the past few months of her depression, which had deepened since Doris's death.

Neither of us knew what we were to do, and that was fine. That was how it had always been. I went to Mum for advice and what she could offer me was reassurance about my abilities, the complications of every possible choice, and the phrase, 'I dunno Chlo.' There was comfort in that acknowledgement. She would support my decisions knowing they were one of many good and bad ones I could make. I wasn't to behave a certain way. I could have said, 'Be brave! You will win the fight with cancer!' and she would have probably told me to fuck off, but she would have understood because one thing she did know was that she didn't know anything, so why should I know what she needed me to say?

And that was the trouble with the death that she would and wouldn't be a part of. That not knowing. I was with her while she died. Her death was almost as mysterious to me as it was to her when she could think and write about it. What was she experiencing? I could only observe her body and my own feelings. From my side, so much love, so much tenderness towards the child in her struggling away, catching breaths. She was hot and silky soft, and I held her hand and lay next to her, not knowing if she knew I was there or could understand that this was the death she had been so desperate to know.

She died on the 28th of April 2016 at four thirty in the morning. It was just as her nurses had told her they could deliver. Mum's pain was managed, her anxiety was too. She was unconscious and at home in her bed, under cashmere.

Did she want company at that moment? I felt she did. I used to tease her about her overuse of the word solitude. She certainly needed to be alone for long stretches of time. But the solitude that she sought so desperately was always dependent on others being there for her to take time away from. She loved to chat, and sing, and was naturally playful. Mum and Ian did lots of that together. In the final weeks of her life, she needed the physical presence of others and, to my surprise, she told me that her main regret was not making more good friends and spending time with people having interesting conversations. She was pretty high when she said that, but her need at that point was obvious. When Doris died it felt to me that she needed it to be a personal and solitary experience. Company during those final days seemed like an intrusion. With Mum, I had the opposite feeling, that she was scared and didn't want to be alone. But, who knows.

I avoided reading *In Gratitude* after she died. I read some of the articles when they were published in the *London Review of Books*, mostly the ones that weren't about her treatment. I wonder if I would have read the book if I hadn't agreed to do this afterword. Probably not for years. I was uncomfortable, even quite annoyed, with Mum for exposing herself and her thoughts about Doris and Peter. I've always been very private and my instinct is to say 'Shhh.' She used to joke that I was Saffy to her Edina from the TV comedy, *Absolutely Fabulous*. That was true enough for her to make the joke. For me, her articles were another layer of complication during her illness. For her, it was what made it easier. Fair enough.

In her first chapter, when she hears the diagnosis, Mum asks, 'Will I suffer in silence . . . or will I refuse to go gentle and make an almighty fuss?' She did a bit of both. Mum hated complaining about the physical difficulties of her illnesses, and whenever she mentioned them she always apologised for being a nuisance and for going on and on, when she never actually did. The fuss was, for me, her fury. My god she was hard to handle. She was so tough. She fought: Doris, her mother, me, Ian, her friends, her nurses, her readers, everyone, with all her might and, crucially, with considerable humour. It wasn't her battling the cancer, fibrosis, or death, but finding the best way to engage with her situation and to understand it.

Of course, the writing process did that too. The most important thing was to try to make the unknown known or at least to create enough of something to observe and engage with. How else could she get some control when she didn't know what time of the day it was or how to move her fingers with enough precision to type a word? She would ring me up while I was in the playground with my children to ask where she was and what day it was. Was she in Spain? There were bruises, black eyes, constant falls, broken bones, terrifying delusions, on top of a deep and grinding depression. During the later stages of her illness, when we came for lunch after not seeing her for weeks because Rosie had chickenpox, she made her entrance by falling into the kitchen, Ian and her legs unable to hold her up. Her body was totally transformed by a steroid-induced 'fat suit', as she called it.

I explained calmly to Louis that Granjen had 'wobbly legs' but the brutality and tragedy of her situation was obvious to him and all of us, especially Mum. The descriptions of her illnesses and the medication's side effects in the book are pretty tame, controlled, some-times humorous. Quite different to her day-to-day experience of them. Her tweets are rawer, and many of them painful to read.

So, during all this, that spirit of revolt helped. In that stance, the embodiment of the fleeting teenage look she describes in the book, she was the self she needed to be. She *was* 'granite', but the granite could fall to dust in a moment. It was hard to know which side you would get. Mum had both states in her already, but the depression, the many pills she was given and withdrawing from, along with the morphine she always kept by her side, made both parts more pronounced.

I may not have felt comfortable with her making her (our) situation so public, but I also admired her open-ness. That refusal to disguise anything by making it more pleasant and inoffensive helped me a great deal. There were no niceties about her illness. We didn't ignore it or pretend that she would be okay. Mum and I often discussed the fact she would die soon, how she felt about it, how I would cope, how I would talk to her grandchildren about her, and she found that relieving. We both did. The writing was part of it. And what brilliant writing it is. Even when she was mad as a bat and her style changed – perhaps a touch more vicious, looser and absurd – it was still astonishingly good.

The parts of the book that have me in tears are the vulnerable bits. Like when she describes her depression in the 1980s, which was essentially about not writing, and Doris told her she could write about her interesting life and someone else could smooth out her prose. I can imagine that happening, and the dissolution, as well as the determination that followed it.

I often felt what she wrote about Doris was true to Mum's experience, but didn't give Doris enough opportunity to be just as fucked-up as Mum. I told Mum so, and she agreed. Doris was flawed, Mum was flawed. Both were damaged by their childhoods and both were just as independent, determined and ruthless when they needed to be. I remember being privy to that anger she talks about when approaching Doris's house. Once we were there it was civil. Tea, cake, politics, but never any mention of each other's work. I think, though, that Doris had a lot of respect for Mum, and was proud of her. I will always remember arriving for tea with Mum towards the end of Doris's life, and seeing Doris's eyes light up and her arms reach out to hold her hands. I honestly don't think I had seen her so thrilled by the presence of someone. She laughed and laughed in her company. Mum really woke Doris up.

Doris and Peter had excruciating final years. I looked after their household, their finances, helped with many medical emergencies, and was generally available for them. I had been very close to Doris, and our relationship was far less complicated than it had been with Mum. I felt the latter period was private, and Peter should be left in peace by Mum, Doris, whoever. Mum, though, was a writer, and you don't censor them. Suggest, but don't censor.

I did try once. I felt one line in her memoir was particularly hard for me to ignore. She wrote that none of the people waiting outside ITU for Peter, including me, had any warmth for him. My feelings about Peter are mixed, but warmth is in there. I hated reading it in the *London Review of Books* and said I would prefer it if she rewrote that line for the book. All hell broke loose. She 'was a *writer*'; she could write what she bloody well wanted and if I didn't like it, well that was my problem. The lack of warmth was her idea of what we all experienced and she had a right to put it down. A few minutes later she changed the sentence. I think after I read it to her and she realised it wasn't a particularly good line anyway. We sat together on her bed and she dictated something else in an instant, which captured the complexity much better. Changing a line of her work at that stage brought on a flood of paranoia, and made the granite world she needed to believe in collapse for a while. She then raged and said all sorts of things which she would have regretted had she the capacity to remember them.

When I visited the following week the fury had gone, and she was in an entirely different mood. She said that she wanted me to write the final chapter of the book, and thought it was very important I should. She knew she wouldn't be able to finish the Doris and Peter section as thoroughly as she would have liked. She wanted me to write my thoughts, uncensored, about her and her illness and my experience with Doris and Peter. She felt her story was also mine and that the final years of Doris and Peter's lives involved us both. I don't want to go into that time, so this afterword is the compromise.

It was a very moving gesture, and a good example of how generous Mum could be. Most of the time she was incredibly thoughtful and considerate of my feelings, my children's feelings, my partner's and, of course, Ian's. She could think herself into anyone's mind, which is why she could attack with such precision when she felt threatened, but it also meant she was able to be the most kind and caring person I have known.

She wanted *In Gratitude* to be dedicated to her grandchildren, Louis and Rosie. The book was rushed to publication so that Mum could hold a copy before she died. As she forgot most things during that period, the intention didn't get through in time for the publication of the hardback. But it did make sense. She was delighted by her grandchildren, and seeing them was an effective medicine. The side effect, though, was the pain of thinking of what she would miss and that they wouldn't know her. It's true, they have lost so much. Louis loved her deeply. Rosie, almost one when she died, enjoyed rolling around her. Mum was surprised at her uncomplicated love for them, and felt pride at creating what she thought was a good mum (me). She said I was better at it than she was. I'm not sure that's true, although I can imagine her worrying constantly about not managing it, which I wouldn't have the energy to do. She often pictured me drugged and dead at twenty-five, just as Doris imagined she would be.

Mum sometimes gave me the experience of what it was like being with her own mother by blasting me with her terror and anger when my life didn't fit with hers (getting us late for school by not finding my shoes, something like that). I was always aware, though, that she was being taken over, and that her calmer more solid self was around and loved me. We were always close. Seeing her arms around Louis and Rosie, and the loving words and tenderness she gave them towards the end when she knew she would soon not have many more opportunities, was very painful to witness. However, it also gave me an inkling of her ability to love with a great strength, and how lucky I am for having that. There was certainty in that part of her, and I think her recognition of that helped her to stay alive, and to write.

So now what is left is her books. Doris's books. Stuff around. Like the multicoloured shawl on the chair in my study, knitted by Mum shortly before her diagnosis. There are photos there taken by Roger, my dad. One with his trainer in the corner of a grey cobbled beach, god knows where, probably in the early eighties. Another, sunnier, of Jewish graves at Kraków which Dad gave to Doris. On the shelf is a pressed leaf with the words 'For Doris Lessing!' and then her addition, 'For Chloe!' underneath. Doris and Peter's record player, which once sat on their green living room floor, is now under a pile of photos and albums that need sorting. I don't remember it ever being used, it must have been for parties long ago. I put on Louis Armstrong during the final year of Doris's life. Mum and Doris both sat quietly smiling, pulled back to the 1960s for three minutes of 'Tea for Two' until Doris waved her hand to signal, 'enough', or, 'too much'. I would have liked it to have gone on and on. I am sentimental. I have a feeling Mum agreed with Doris.